Overcoming Common Problems Series

D0300260

Overcoming Common Problems Series

Overcoming Common Problems

Your Guide for the Cancer Journey

Cancer and its treatment

MARK GREENER

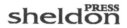

First published in Great Britain in 2018

Sheldon Press
36 Causton Street
London SW1P 4ST
www.sheldonpress.co.uk

British Library Cataloguing-in-Publication Data
A catalogue record for this book is available from the British Library

ISBN 978-1-84709-439-1
eBook ISBN 978-1-84709-440-7

Typeset by Fakenham Prepress Solutions, Fakenham, Norfolk NR21 8NN
First printed in Great Britain by Ashford Colour Press
Subsequently digitally reprinted in Great Britain

eBook by Fakenham Prepress Solutions, Fakenham, Norfolk NR21 8NN

Produced on paper from sustainable forests

To Rose, Yasmin, Rory and Ophelia

Contents

Note to the reader

This is not a medical book and is not intended to replace advice from your doctor, cancer team or other healthcare professional. Consult your pharmacist, doctor or cancer team if you believe you have any of the symptoms described or if you think you might need medical help.

Introduction

Some 2 million people in the UK – about 1 in every 33 – are cancer survivors. Doctors expect this figure to reach 4 million by 2030.[1] Advances in screening, diagnosis and treatment mean that more and more people with cancer are cured or survive for longer. According to Macmillan Cancer Support, people now live nearly ten times longer after their cancer diagnosis than they did 40 years ago. In the early 1970s, half of people diagnosed with cancer in England and Wales lived for at least a year. By 2007, half of people with cancer lived for at least six years. Today, experts predict that half of people diagnosed with cancer in England and Wales in 2010–11 will survive for at least ten years.[1]

Indeed, the prognosis for certain cancers is better than that for some other common diseases. For example, between half and up to more than 9 in 10 (50–99 per cent) of men with prostate cancer, and at least three-quarters (73–89 per cent) of women with breast cancer, live for more than five years. By way of comparison, half (50 per cent) of people who have a stroke and about 3 in 5 (62 per cent) of those who develop heart failure live for at least five years.[2]

Reduction in cancer-related deaths

Since the early 1970s, the number of people dying from cancer has fallen by about a fifth (22 per cent) in females and by about a tenth (8 per cent) in men, according to Cancer Research UK. The improved prospects have been even more dramatic in some cancers. For instance, the number of children under 15 years of age who die from cancer in Great Britain fell by about a third (32 per cent) between 1994/1996 and 2013/2015. Chemotherapy – an important class of anti-cancer drugs – is responsible for most of the reduction in cancer-related deaths among children.

Indeed, about 403,000 fewer people in the UK are expected to die from cancer over the next 20 years because of improved detection, diagnosis and treatments than if mortality remained the same as it is today. Cancer Research UK estimate that, compared to 2014, deaths from cancer will drop by about a seventh (15 per cent) by

2035. The prospects for some cancers will probably improve by much more. For instance, Cancer UK estimates that deaths from bowel cancer will fall by about a quarter (23 per cent) by 2035.

Catching cancer early – such as when it is still small enough for surgeons to remove totally – remains the best chance for a cure. Nevertheless, there are grounds for cautious optimism even for some advanced and metastatic cancers (malignancies that have spread to another part of the body). In the early 1970s, for example, 19 in 20 men with metastatic testicular cancers died, usually within 1 year of diagnosis, according to the National Institutes of Health in the USA. Modern treatments cure 4 in 5 metastatic testicular cancers. Moreover, the cancer team can draw on a growing array of modern medical advances – often at biology's cutting edge – to help you live as full a life as possible, for as long as possible. Even if the cancer is incurable, the cancer team might be able to control the malignancy, sometimes for many years.

Long-term health

Being given the all-clear from cancer doesn't necessarily mean your health problems are over. The physical and psychological effects of cancer can linger, sometimes for several years. Radiotherapy and chemotherapy can also cause late effects that might emerge many years after treatment ends. Even a decade after being diagnosed with the malignancy, survivors of breast and colorectal cancer were still more likely to see their GP than people who had not had cancer.[3]

Certain physical symptoms may not arise until months or even years after cancer treatment ends, such as osteoporosis (brittle bones) following endocrine (hormonal) therapies, heart disease after certain types of chemotherapy or radiotherapy, and malignancies caused by the treatment of the initial cancer.[1] Macmillan Cancer Support notes that, in the UK, 1 in 4 people faces poor health or disability after cancer treatment ends. Lifestyle changes and active management by the cancer team can often help lift this long-term burden.

Cancer – a common concern

Cancer is probably the most feared disease. Indeed, more than half (55 per cent) of us worry about cancer occasionally or sometimes, according to researchers who interviewed 2,048 people in England between 18 and 70 years old. The study, presented at the 2016 National Cancer Research Institute conference, also found that about 1 in 14 (7 per cent) of us worries about cancer often or very often.

There's often good reason for our fears. After all, half of us who were born after 1960 will probably be diagnosed with cancer at some point, according to Cancer Research UK. So the risk of developing cancer is about the same as correctly calling 'heads' when flipping a coin, and everyone knows a friend, family member or colleague who has had cancer. Doctors diagnosed 356,860 new cancers in the UK during 2014. In other words, doctors give someone a diagnosis of cancer every two minutes or so. During 2014, 163,444 people died from cancer: 1 death from cancer every 3 minutes.

Cancer is also increasingly common (partly because we are, on average, living longer), which helps fuel the fears. Cancer Research UK says that since the late 1970s, the number of cancer cases has risen by two-fifths (37 per cent) in females and by almost a fifth in males (17 per cent). If current trends continue, the number of cancer cases could rise by two-fifths (40 per cent) between 2014 and 2035.[4] But it's not all bad news.

Improvements across the board

All areas of cancer care – from screening to palliative care – have improved dramatically over recent years. For example, the outcomes for surgical procedures have been improved by technological advances, better aftercare and improved rehabilitation. These advances do not just mean that the operation is more likely to remove all the cancer than in the past; they also cause less collateral damage to healthy tissue. So the cosmetic appearance is better and the operation is less likely to have effects on your health (complications).

For example, advances in robotic surgery allow surgeons to perform incredibly delicate operations, such as removing cancers from the prostate gland, which is surrounded by a network of important nerves.[3] Robotic surgery seems to reduce the number of men who develop some complications commonly linked to conventional prostate surgery, such as lifelong erectile dysfunction and incontinence.

Meanwhile, radiotherapists can now target X-rays to the tumour with unprecedented accuracy. Cancers are not regular solid balls of cells. They are irregularly shaped and vary in density. Sophisticated computer programs vary the focus and intensity of the beam of X-rays to match the cancer's shape and density. Treating a cancer always means treading a fine line between killing as many malignant cells as possible and avoiding damage to healthy tissue that causes short-term (acute) and persistent (chronic) adverse events. These new programs maximize the number of cancer cells killed while limiting the damage to the healthy tissue. So the radiotherapist might be able to deliver a higher dose of X-rays to the tumour and less to the surrounding tissue. This, in turn, increases the chance of a good outcome with fewer complications.

Hardly a day goes by without a new study elucidating some fresh insight into cancer biology, such as how a tumour emerges, grows and spreads. This increasing understanding of cancer biology is revealing new targets in critical pathways that drive the malignancy's development and, in turn, inspiring innovative new treatments. Indeed, in 2016, the European Society for Medical Oncology estimated that 225 new cancer treatments would be introduced by 2020.[5] Even if they do not all reach the clinic, the figure underscores the remarkable pace of innovation.

For example, some older cancer drugs are relatively indiscriminate, killing malignant cells but also harming healthy tissue, hence the hair loss and other 'classic' side effects of chemotherapy. Doctors can mix-and-match the chemotherapy drugs in the cocktail and increase or decrease the dose of one or more medicines, but in general, 'one size fits all'. Modern cancer drugs are increasingly tailored to your particular cancer at that stage, often based on insights from genetic studies (called 'personalized medicine').

A genetic disease

As we will see, cancer is predominately a genetic disease. Your genetic code is a series of instructions that control your body's structure, appearance and function. Some genes, for example, determine whether you are naturally a blonde, brunette or redhead.

Others partly determine your height, and other genes determine the way cells divide in order to, for instance, repair damage in the body or replace old cells. In many cases, several genes interact to exert their effects.

Cells are the building blocks of our body – and they are highly specialized. The skin cells that touch this book are very different from the light-sensitive cells at the back of your eye that detect the words on the page. The light-sensitive cells are very different from the nerve cells in the brain that interpret what the words mean.

Too many cells – even if they are not malignant – and too few can harm health and well-being, so a complex network of signals controls the production of new cells and the destruction of old ones. But changes to the genetic code – mutations – can send abnormal signals to the cells. This means cells begin to divide out of control – one of the hallmarks of cancer. Other mutations drive the cancer's progression, such as when the tumour invades the surrounding healthy tissue or fragments break off and spread to other parts of the body (metastases). Mutations are also responsible for changes that mean cancer treatments may stop working (resistance).

Increasingly, however, these mutations are also cancer's Achilles heel. For example, researchers can now look at the pattern of mutations in the genetic code of a cancer and sometimes use these to develop new drugs. For example, by binding to a protein produced by the mutated gene, the drug might be able to stop the cancer from dividing. The drug, however, will work only if the cancer has 'switched on' (expresses) that gene.

The cancer team

During your cancer journey you will draw on the expertise of a range of healthcare professionals. The team's multidisciplinary membership will depend on your needs but typically will include:

- a surgeon with expertise in your cancer: operating for head and neck cancer is very different from removing a breast tumour, for example;
- a pathologist who looks at cancer samples to diagnose the malignancy and assess the tumour's characteristics – so the pathologist might assess how aggressive the cancer is and, in some cases, use the cancer's biology to tailor treatment;

- a radiologist, who might use high-tech imaging to look inside your body and deliver X-rays to treat the cancer;
- an oncologist – a doctor specializing in cancer treatment – might discuss which drugs you need based on the cancer's characteristics, any other diseases you might have and how well you are generally;
- nurse specialists who have particular expertise in cancer care.

In other cases, the team might include a dietician or speech and language therapist, who can help if you have difficulties eating or with speech. If you develop emotional or mental health issues, the team might include a counsellor or psychiatrist. Also, you will probably see your GP more often than you did before you were diagnosed with cancer.

In many cases you will receive high-tech cancer treatments. Do not worry if you find the details difficult to understand at first. Some new treatments are highly sophisticated scientifically and at the very edge of our biological understanding – even non-specialist healthcare professionals can have difficulty understanding how they work. So always ask your cancer team and patient groups, such as Cancer Research UK and Macmillan Cancer Support, if you do not understand something or have questions.

A personal journey

Broadly, a cancer journey has three stages.

- **Soon after diagnosis** the cancer team tries to cure or limit the damage caused by the malignancy. This might involve surgery, radiotherapy, medicines or, for most people, a mixture of approaches. Although you might feel that your life is in your cancer team's hands, you can still deal with side effects, remain positive and understand what the cancer team is doing and why. Do not underestimate the importance of these steps: they give cancer treatment the best chance of working, help limit collateral damage and maximize your quality of life.
- **The recovery phase** during which you get over the worst effects of treatment and restore your physical and mental well-being. The cancer team will monitor you to detect any relapses.
- **The maintenance phase** during which you take steps to prevent

or delay a recurrence, prevent additional malignancies and reduce the risk of other diseases.[6]

This book focuses on the first of these stages and if the cancer recurs. My book *The Holistic Guide for Cancer Survivors* places more emphasis on the second two stages. There is some overlap, however, especially when we consider the steps you can take to deal with effects of the cancer and its treatment.

The bravery people show when they face cancer never ceases to amaze me. Nevertheless, your cancer journey will be deeply personal, often difficult and at times frightening. Cancer is enigmatic, capricious and unpredictable. Despite advances in imaging and genetics, no one can precisely define what will happen (your prognosis). No one can accurately predict the severity of side effects or long-term complications or the extent to which the cancer and its treatment will disrupt your life. Your cancer team offers educated guesses based on scientific data, but there are countless cases where patients have defied their doctors' expectations.

Likewise, no one can guarantee that the general information and suggestions in this book will definitely work for or apply to you. *These suggestions do not replace the advice from your cancer team, which is tailored to you, your cancer and your circumstances.* Always contact your GP or cancer team if you feel unwell or think your disease is getting worse, even if it is between your routine appointments.

A note about references

It is impossible to cite all the medical and scientific studies that I used to write this book (apologies to anyone whose work I missed). I've highlighted certain papers to illustrate important points and themes. You can find a summary of most of the papers by visiting the website: <www.ncbi.nlm.nih.gov/pubmed>. Some full papers are available online free or at a reduced rate for patients. Larger libraries might stock or allow you to access some medical journals. Some of the papers might seem rather erudite if you do not have a medical or biological background, but do not let that put you off. If you feel that you do not understand something, please ask your GP, pharmacist, cancer team or a helpline run by a charity, such as Cancer Research UK or Macmillan Cancer Support.

1

Cells out of control

I'm not, literally, the same man I was a few years ago. My cells live for, on average, seven to ten years. A cell's lifespan varies from about three to four months for my 30 trillion red blood cells to more than 50 years for some heart cells. In addition, I constantly repair, renew and replenish my long-lived cells: I replace all the water in my body every few weeks, for instance.[7, 8]

We produce new cells to replace old and damaged tissues. Too few or too many cells can upset the body's normal finely balanced function. So a complex control system fine-tunes the destruction and production of cells. For example, the immune system – which protects us from invading bacteria, viruses and parasites – destroys some damaged cells. Meanwhile, certain chemical messengers promote cell division, while others reduce it. Some messengers trigger cells to self-destruct. Such checks and balances mean that, when we are healthy, the number of cells we produce balances the number we lose.

Cancers unbalance this system. Certain malignancies, for example, evade destruction by the immune system. In some cancers, the messengers no longer stimulate worn-out cells to self-destruct. In other malignancies, more cells are produced than are destroyed.

Indeed, in many ways a cancer exaggerates the activities of normal cells. All cells divide, but cancer cells often divide more prolifically than healthy cells. All cells are vulnerable to damage by, for example, chemotherapy or radiotherapy, but cancer cells are more susceptible (a difference that allows doctors to target the cancer cells while limiting, as far as possible, damage to healthy tissue). All cells adapt to changes in the body, but cancer cells are genetically unstable and so adapt more rapidly (which is why cancers can become resistant to some drugs).

Cells, tissues and organs

- **Cells** are your body's building blocks. A bacterium, spermatozoa or ovum (human egg) and the amoeba you might remember from biology class are single cells. You need a microscope to see most single cells. Nerve cells that run from the spinal cord to a toe can be a metre long but are very thin. An ovum is about the size of a sharp pencil point. It's the only human cell you can see with the naked eye.[8]
- **Tissues** are organized collections of cells between a single cell and an organ. Most organs consist of several tissues.
- **Organs** are self-contained, organized collections of cells with one or more functions. The lungs, for example, are collections of cells that exchange toxic carbon dioxide for the oxygen that keeps us alive. The liver is a collection of cells that, among other actions, removes waste. The heart is a collection of cells that pumps blood.

Abnormal cells

Broadly, a cancer's development takes place in three stages: initiation, promotion and progression. Here are examples of what happens in each stage.

- **Initiation** Even a single exposure to certain carcinogens can trigger a mutation, which is passed on to new generations when the cell divides. At this stage (initiation) the cell looks and acts normally.[2]
- **Promotion**, the next stage, can require exposure to another carcinogen or mutation that gives the cancer a growth advantage over the surrounding healthy tissue (the cancer may divide more rapidly, for example). In the 1940s, for instance, researchers found that about 1 in 20 mice (5 per cent) treated with a chemical called benzopyrene developed cancers, but this increased to 4 in 5 (80 per cent) when the mice were also treated with croton oil, a chemical carcinogen extracted from the seeds of a tree cultivated in India. Croton oil promoted cancer but, on its own, did not cause malignancies.[2]
- **Progression** When the cancer enters this phase it begins to show the hallmark abnormalities of a malignancy (see below). At this stage, carcinogens can cause mutations that drive progression,

but mutations can emerge spontaneously – as mentioned before, cancers are genetically very unstable (see also page 28).[2]

Transformation into a cancer

As the cancer moves from initiation to progression, the cell undergoes marked changes in structure, appearance and function. The transformation of a healthy cell into a cancer begins when the number of cells in an organ or tissue increases. These cells look normal under a microscope. Doctors call this stage hyperplasia.

Over time, the cells begin to look abnormal, but they are still not cancerous. Doctors call this stage dysplasia. Hyperplasia and dysplasia do not always develop into cancer. Sometimes hyperplasia and dysplasia progress no further. Sometimes the body's innate healing abilities reverse the abnormality and restore normal healthy tissue. Sometimes, however, dysplastic cells develop into a malignancy.

Cancer cells look profoundly abnormal and no longer perform their normal functions. As the cancer grows, abnormal cells replace more and more healthy tissue. Eventually, the organ cannot compensate. Symptoms emerge and the organ begins to fail. That is why, unfortunately, cancers can kill. To understand cancer, we need to look at how cells divide.

Well- or poorly differentiated cancers

You may read or hear the cancer team talk about well- or poorly differentiated cancers.

- **Well-differentiated cancers** closely resemble the organization, shape and appearance of the tissues in which they arose. So a well-differentiated breast cancer looks similar to normal breast tissue.
- **Poorly differentiated cancers** grow rapidly and look very different from the tissue of origin, so are 'more abnormal' than a well-differentiated malignancy.

The degree of differentiation can influence survival. For example, almost all (95 per cent) women with well-differentiated breast cancer are still alive five years after their diagnosis. This falls to half (50 per cent) of those with poorly differentiated tumours.[2]

Cell division

We need to replace damaged and old tissues to stay healthy, so our cells divide into two identical 'daughter cells'. Each daughter cell then becomes specialized (differentiation). For example, we need to replace the 30,000 skin cells we lose each minute.[7] So cells in the bottom layer of the skin split into two. These then differentiate, becoming skin – and not liver – cells. Most cells in the human body are not actively dividing (proliferating) – they are 'quiescent'. The exceptions are rapidly renewing tissues, such as skin and bone marrow, which produces blood cells.[9] This difference in proliferation influences side effects from many cancer treatments.

The cell cycle (see Figure 1.1) refers to the series of events that occurs as the cell divides, including duplicating all the cell's contents that keep it alive and healthy and copying the genetic code. A change in the genetic code (such as a mutation) – as cancer demonstrates – can be serious. So sensors, called checkpoints, control the cell's progression through each phase. These checkpoints maintain the correct order of the stages in the cell cycle. The sensors also control the cell's movement from one phase to the next, diverting damaged or abnormal cells until they can be repaired or destroyed, usually by a process called apoptosis (see box 'Necrosis and apoptosis').[9]

For example, a protein called p53 is a checkpoint that normally prevents cells with damaged DNA from becoming cancerous.[10] Numerous stresses can cause p53 to halt the cell cycle. These include well-known carcinogens – such as tobacco smoke and ultraviolet radiation in sunlight and tanning beds – but also more subtle changes, such as low levels of oxygen and glucose in the cell.[10] As we will see in Chapter 2, mutations to the genes that produce p53 and some other checkpoints are common in many cancers.

The changes to the checkpoints mean that cancer cells are essentially immortal: the body no longer destroys old and damaged cells. For example, biologists use HeLa cells grown in the laboratory to investigate cancer and in other experiments. The billions of HeLa cells in laboratories around the world derive from a fragment of cervical cancer taken from a woman in 1951. In contrast, normal human cells grown in the laboratory (called 'cell culture') split 60 or 70 times before dying.[2, 11] As their lifespans illustrate, cancer cells and healthy cells differ fundamentally.

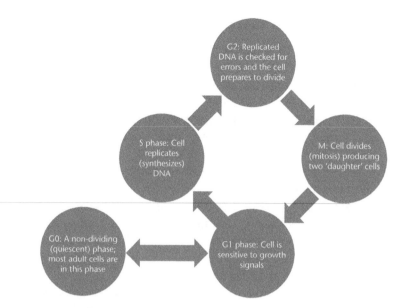

Figure 1.1 The cell cycle, simplified

Necrosis and apoptosis

Cells can die in one of two ways, which biologists call necrosis and apoptosis. Necrosis usually follows damage to the body, such as injury, infection and toxins. A thin membrane surrounds each cell. In necrosis, damage to the cell membrane means that the contents leak out, triggering inflammation. Normally, inflammation is an important weapon in our immune defences: it helps fight infection and encourages healing. Too much inflammation, however, can damage the surrounding tissues. Indeed, many cancers trigger excessive inflammation, which promotes their growth.[2]

Apoptosis is 'controlled cell death' that does not trigger inflammation or immune responses.[2] During apoptosis, which generally takes 30–120 minutes,[2] the membrane that surrounds each cell remains intact. In the 'sac' formed by the membrane, the cell's contents are gradually broken down and removed, such as by being swallowed by certain white blood cells. In addition to removing old and damaged cells, apoptosis helps our bodies form in the womb, removing the web of skin between our fingers and toes (in most people), and hollowing out blood vessels and other tubes.[10] In other words, controlled cell death is essential for life.

A long time coming

Most cancers have been growing for years before they are large enough to cause symptoms. For example, on average, a breast cancer cell divides every 100 days. A breast cancer of 1 cm across, the size you might feel or see on a mammogram, contains about a million cells[12] and has probably been growing for between five and six years. Some cancers grow so slowly that people die with, rather than from, the malignancy. Most men of 80 years of age show cancer cells in their prostate gland, for example, but 1 in 25 die from prostate cancer.[2]

Likewise, an infection with hepatitis C virus (HCV) takes decades to develop into liver cancer. The immune systems of up to a fifth (20 per cent) of people clear HCV naturally within six months of contracting the virus. Many of the remainder never develop signs or symptoms, though they can still infect others.[13]

However, at least a quarter of people with chronic HCV develop cirrhosis (scarring of the liver) within 30–40 years of infection.[13] Between 1 in 100 and 1 in 25 people with cirrhosis due to HCV develop liver cancer each year.[14] This long lag-time and the fact that more than one 'hit' is usually needed to produce a cancer offers the chance to prevent some malignancies either by lifestyle changes (such as stopping smoking or drinking alcohol) or by screening (see page 11).

Any cell can turn cancerous. Oncologists recognize more than 200 malignancies and often there are several subtypes. Some cancers emerge in only a handful of people each year, while others, malignancies of the breast, lung, prostate and bowel, for example, account for about half of cancers (54 per cent) and cancer deaths (46 per cent).

The same cancer's characteristics can differ dramatically from person to person. There are at least four main subtypes of breast cancer, for instance, each caused by different abnormalities[15] and each with a different prognosis (outlook) and sometimes treatments. Cancers affecting the same organ also vary depending on their cell or tissue of origin. Basal cell carcinoma, squamous cell carcinoma, melanoma and Merkel cell carcinoma are all skin cancers, but arise from different cells, so they have different characteristics, prognoses and treatments. That is one reason why I doubt there will ever be a single cure for cancer: each malignancy, each subtype and even each stage will probably need a different cure.

What's in a name?

Cancers tend to be named after their tissue of origin. Here are some examples.

- A thin layer of epithelial cells lines many parts of the body, including the skin, intestines and lungs. Carcinomas are cancers that arise from epithelial cells.
- Connective tissue supports, connects and separates other tissues and organs. Sarcomas refers to cancers beginning in connective tissue, such as cartilage, muscle, tendon or bone. Sarcomas make up 1 in 100 (1 per cent) of all cancers in adults and there are at least 50 subtypes.[2]
- Lymphomas arise in lymph glands or other organs of the lymphatic system.
- Leukaemia refers to cancers of white blood cells, which normally protect us from infections. Blood cancers do not normally form solid tumours.
- Melanoma arises in cells that give our skin its colour.

What is lymph?

Lymph is a clear, milky or yellowish fluid that bathes our tissues and contains the white blood cells that fight infections and cancers. That is why your lymph nodes – such as the 'glands' under your chin and in your armpits – might swell when you have an infection or you are fighting cancer. Your lymph glands might also swell as invading cancer cells grow inside the node. So the cancer team might surgically remove or irradiate (treat with radiotherapy) lymph nodes near the cancer.

Primary and secondary cancers

Doctors call the original tumour the 'primary cancer'. Cancerous cells can spread from the original tumour to other parts of the body where they can form 'secondary cancers', also called 'metastases'. So a doctor will refer to, for instance, metastatic prostate cancer. In general, advanced cancer means a cure is, unfortunately, unlikely. Most people with advanced cancer have metastases.

Doctors distinguish 'second primary cancers' from secondary cancers. A second primary cancer refers to a new primary cancer (*not* a metastasis) in a person who has already had a malignancy. So a skin cancer caused by too much sun in a person who survived breast cancer is a second primary malignancy. Sometimes chemotherapy or radiotherapy – both of which damage DNA – may trigger a second primary cancer many years after treatment ends.

Occasionally (3–5 per cent of cancers), identifying the primary cancer of someone with a metastatic malignancy can prove difficult. Sometimes the cancer is too small. In other cases the cancer might have regressed at its site of origin. Doctors call this 'a cancer of unknown primary'. Advances in diagnosis mean that the number of cancers of unknown primary is declining.[2]

Second primary cancers

Occasionally, cancer treatments can lead to a second primary cancer. For example, second leukaemias and lymphomas peak 2–4 years after chemotherapy for Hodgkin's lymphoma ends. The rise in solid cancers – such as breast, colorectal and lung – typically occurs 15–20 years after the diagnosis of Hodgkin's lymphoma.[2] Patients younger than 40 years old treated with radiotherapy or chemotherapy for Hodgkin's lymphoma, non-Hodgkin's lymphoma or testicular cancer are roughly four times more likely than the general public to develop a second primary cancer.[1]

Benign and cancerous tumours

An abnormal accumulation of cells – a tumour or neoplasm – is not always cancerous. Doctors call non-cancerous accumulations of cells 'benign' tumours. Unlike cancers, benign tumours do not invade other tissues or metastasize. When removed by surgeons, most benign tumours do not regrow (called a recurrence) and rarely cause serious health difficulties. Sometimes, however, a benign tumour can press on a nearby area, which might cause symptoms. An acoustic neuroma, for example, arises in the nerve from the ear to the brain and can affect hearing and balance.[16] Some benign tumours in glands can overproduce hormones, which can be harmful to health.[2]

Hallmarks of cancer

Cancer cells show several hallmarks that differentiate them from normal cells. Here are some examples.

- Healthy cells depend on a network of signals that stimulate them to divide and then to stop. Cancer cells are self-sufficient. They do not rely on external signals, so cancers do not stop growing despite signals that tell them to: they avoid apoptosis and do not show signs of age. As mentioned, cancer cells are effectively immortal.
- Cancer cells are able to feed themselves (by growing new blood vessels, for example – see page 77). Some highly effective drugs for certain cancers work by preventing the formation of new blood vessels – a process called angiogenesis.
- Cancers can trigger inflammation and evade destruction by the host's immune system.
- Cancer dysregulates the way cells make energy.
- Importantly, cancers can invade healthy tissue and metastasize.[2]

Spreading cancer around the body

Cancers are malignant – sometimes called invasive. In other words, the cancer can spread into – invade – nearby tissues (see Figure 1.2). Indeed, the term cancer comes from a Greek word meaning crab. Ancient healers felt that a tumour and its blood vessels had a 'crab-like' appearance as it spread into the surrounding tissue.[17]

Cells can break off from the cancer and travel in the blood or lymph system to other parts of the body. These 'circulating cancer cells' are malignant seeds. They can lodge in another tissue and, if the conditions are right, grow into a metastasis. Sometimes the cancer has spread to other parts of the body by the time doctors diagnose the malignancy, which influences prognosis. Almost 9 in 10 (88 per cent) of women with breast cancer of less than 2 cm across that has not spread to lymph nodes at diagnosis live for at least five years. This falls to 1 in 8 (12 per cent) of those with metastatic breast cancer at diagnosis.[2] That is why screening is so important.

The metastasis changes as it adapts to growing in the new organ. The metastasis, however, retains many characteristics of the primary cancer. So a liver metastasis is different from a primary liver cancer. However, liver metastasis from a breast cancer might

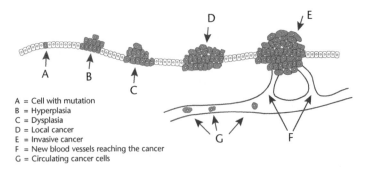

A = Cell with mutation
B = Hyperplasia
C = Dysplasia
D = Local cancer
E = Invasive cancer
F = New blood vessels reaching the cancer
G = Circulating cancer cells

Figure 1.2 The spread of cancer

also differ from the primary cancer. All this makes the treatment of advanced cancer very complicated.

Different cancers, different metastases

Each cancer seems to produce a particular pattern of metastases (see Table 1.1). Symptoms depend on the site of the metastases. Symptoms of a lung metastasis differ from secondary cancer in the brain, for example. The spine is the most common site of metastatic bone tumours, usually in the upper and middle back (the thoracic spine), which can cause spinal cord compression.[3] Lung, breast and kidney cancer as well as melanoma are the malignancies most likely to metastasize to the brain.[2]

The prognosis differs depending on the site of the metastases. In one study, three-quarters (73 per cent) of women with breast

Table 1.1 Common sites of metastases[3]

Primary cancer	Common metastases
Bladder	Brain, lung
Breast	Bone, brain, liver, lung
Colorectal	Liver, lung
Kidney	Bone, brain, lung
Lung	Bone, brain, liver
Melanoma	Brain, liver
Oesophageal	Liver
Pancreatic	Liver
Prostate gland	Bone, brain, lung

cancer and a single metastasis in their skeleton survived for five years. This compared with just over a fifth (22 per cent) of those with a metastasis in an internal organ, such as the liver or lung.[18] Most people with brain metastases, however, die within a month without treatment.[3]

Spinal cord compression

Between 1 in 20 and 1 in 10 (5–10 per cent) people with cancer develop spinal cord compression when a metastasis grows in the bone or surrounding tissue. Spinal cord compression usually causes back pain, often described as band-like discomfort, though of course, back pain can arise from many causes. While diagnosing spinal cord compression can be challenging, a scan usually detects it.

As the pressure on the nerves continues, people might experience a variety of symptoms, such as:

- changes in their senses
- weakness
- pain
- bowel and bladder issues
- sexual difficulties.

The symptoms depend on the site and severity of the compression.

So, if you develop new or worsening back pain, it is worth telling your cancer team as soon as possible. Surgery and radiotherapy can relieve the compression. Early treatment means about 7 in 10 people with spinal cord compression remain mobile, but treatment restores mobility in only 1 in 10 of those with paraplegia (complete or incomplete leg paralysis).[3]

Catching curable cancers

As mentioned, most cancers grow for several years before invading the surrounding tissue. Early detection and rapid treatment offer the best prospect of a cure: surgeons can remove, and so cure, small localized cancers. The aim of screening, therefore, is to detect and treat cervical, breast, prostate and some intestinal malignancies before they are large enough to spread. Screening can be remarkably effective.

- Deaths from cancer of the cervix (the neck of the womb) have decreased by almost three-quarters (71 per cent) in the UK since the early 1970s, largely due to screening.[19]
- Regular cervical screening prevents almost half (about 45 per cent) of cervical cancers in women in their thirties and three-quarters (75 per cent) of those in women in their fifties and sixties.[19]
- Screening detects about 1 in 20 colorectal (bowel) cancers and 3 in 10 breast cancers.[1]
- Deaths from breast cancer in the USA declined by almost a quarter (24 per cent) between 1990 and 2005. Improved chemotherapy probably accounted for half the improvement and screening for the remainder.[17]

Screening can even catch abnormal cells before they turn cancerous. Cervical cancer screening, for example, aims to detect abnormal cells on the surface of the cervix. Doctors grade this 'cervical intra-epithelial neoplasia' (CIN) on a scale of 1 to 3, based on how abnormal the cells look under the microscope and how much of the cervix is affected. CIN is not cancer. Over time, however, between 2 and 3 in every five CIN2 (that is, moderately abnormal) changes return to normal without treatment.[20] Unfortunately, doctors cannot yet predict which CINs will develop into cervical cancers. That is why every woman should attend for screening. Unfortunately, there are no screening tests for many deadly cancers – such as lung, ovary, brain or pancreas – although researchers are working on them.

2

Causes of cancer

As we've seen, in many ways cancer exaggerates normal biology. So, not surprisingly, cancer has always been with us: some bones of dinosaurs and *Homo erectus* – one of our ancestors that lived 1.3–1.8 million years ago – show evidence of tumours.[10] We have also been trying to treat cancer for millennia: Ancient Egyptian medical texts written between 3000 and 1500 BC mention cancer.[10]

Nevertheless, many cancers are part of the price we pay for a modern lifestyle. According to Cancer Research UK, lifestyle factors cause about 2 in 5 cancers (42 per cent). Indeed, with all the scare stories that regularly reach the headlines, you could be forgiven for thinking that almost anything can cause cancer. Over the years, studies have linked cancer to chemicals in food, toys and make-up, air travel, bacon, sausages, chips, burnt toast, and sex . . . the list goes on and on and on.

Hundreds of chemicals have been proved or are likely to cause cancer, at least in cells grown in the laboratory or experimental animals. Often it is not clear if the results apply to humans, yet there's often something to these scare stories. For instance, the higher you travel in the atmosphere, the greater your exposure to cancer-causing cosmic rays. Processed, burnt carbohydrates and, probably, red meat may increase the risk of developing certain malignancies. Also, sex can spread cancer-causing infections.

There are too many potential causes to look at in any detail here, but the following examples illustrate the wide range of cancer risk factors. Doing what you can to tackle these may reduce your risk of a second primary cancer or improve your prospects during cancer treatment.

Radiation

In 1895, a German scientist called Wilhelm Conrad Röntgen accidentally discovered X-rays while experimenting with vacuum tubes.

A week later, Röntgen took the first X-ray image (radiograph) of his wife's hand, showing her bones and wedding ring. The discovery revolutionized medical diagnosis.

The radiographic pioneers soon realized that X-rays can cause burns and skin reactions. In 1902, for example, an X-ray technician developed a sore on his hand. This evolved into the cancer that killed him four years later.[21, 22] The first reports of leukaemia among people working with radioactive materials emerged in 1911.[22] Radiation destroyed the bone marrow of Marie Curie, who won two Nobel Prizes for her pioneering work on radioactivity, leaving her permanently anaemic. Curie died from leukaemia in 1934.[17]

Today, exposure to radioactive material – which scientists call ionizing radiation – probably causes about 1 in 50 cancers in the UK. The risk of getting some blood cancers is especially high: radiation causes about 1 in 13 cases of leukaemia in women and 1 in 15 in men.[22] Children are between 2 and 5 times more sensitive to radiation than adults.[3]

Radon gas

The nuclear accidents that happened at Chernobyl, Three Mile Island and Fukushima highlight the environmental impact of radioactivity, but we're exposed to natural radiation as we go about our daily lives. For instance, radon gas is a natural form of radioactivity that accounts for about half our total exposure to radiation (you can learn more, including what the local levels are, at: <www.ukradon.org>).

Radon arises from deposits of granite, which contains uranium. As the uranium decays, it releases radioactive radon gas. When the soil overlying the granite is porous, the radon can escape and cause cancer in people who live nearby. The risk of lung cancer is 14 per cent higher if someone lives in a house for 30 years with a high level of radon gas (such as 150 Becquerels/m³ compared to the average indoor rate of 20 Becquerels/m³ in the UK).[2]

Other natural sources of radiation – including the cosmic rays linked to cancer in airline staff – account for about a third (35 per cent) of our exposure to radiation. Radiation received during diagnosis and medical procedures – excluding radiotherapy – account for most of the remainder (15 per cent).[22]

Viruses

The first hospital specializing in cancer opened in Reims, France, in 1779. The hospital lay some way outside the town: physicians worried that cancer was contagious.[10] Outside a few exceptional circumstances (see box 'Catching a cancer'), cancer does not spread directly, but some infections increase the risk of developing certain cancers. Indeed, infections seem to cause about 1 in 7 cancers worldwide (15 per cent):

- viruses cause about 1 in 9 cancers (11 per cent);
- bacteria cause about 1 in 25 cancers (4 per cent);
- helminths (parasitic worms) cause about 1 in 1,000 cancers (0.1 per cent)[2] – a parasitic worm living in freshwater in sub-tropical and tropical regions can trigger bladder cancer, for example; [2]
- overall, infections cause about 1 in 27 cancers in the UK.[23]

Some viruses are remarkably potent carcinogens. For example, up to 40 per cent of men infected with chronic hepatitis B virus (HBV) develop hepatocellular carcinoma, which accounts for three-quarters of liver cancers. A study from Taiwan reported that men with chronic HBV were 98 times more likely to develop hepatocellular carcinoma than those without HBV. By contrast, smoking seems to increase the risk of lung cancer 17 times.[2] You can catch HBV from blood and other infected body fluids. If you are at high risk of catching the virus, you can be vaccinated against HBV – speak to your GP or check out the NHS Choices website at: <www.nhs.uk/pages/home.aspx>.

HPV: more than cervical cancer

Each year, thousands of girls in the UK receive a vaccine that protects against human papilloma virus (HPV), which seems to cause 1 in 20 cancers (4.8 per cent) worldwide. Cervical cancer is the best-known malignancy linked to HPV, but the virus also causes some cancers of the vulva, vagina, penis, anus and some head and neck cancers.[2]

Biologists have identified more than 200 types of HPV.[24] More than 40 of these potentially infect the area around the anus and genitals, and 14 types of HPV can cause cervical cancers.[25] Two

Catching a cancer

Very occasionally it is possible to catch a cancer directly. Normally cancer cells, although immortal, die when the 'host' (the patient, for example) passes away. In a handful of cases, however, the cancer can take on a life of its own and pass directly from animal to animal. For example, a facial tumour is driving the Tasmanian devil, a marsupial, to the edge of extinction and canine transmissible venereal tumour, as its name suggests, usually spreads when dogs mate. In both cases, the cancer cells spread from animal to animal and trigger the malignancy in the recipients.

There do not seem to be any similar malignancies in humans, but cancer cells in transplanted organs can occasionally cause malignancies in the recipient. Cancer cells can also cross the placenta from mother to child.[2] These are very unusual cases, however.

types – HPV 16 and 18 – seem to account for approximately 7 in 10 (70 per cent) of cervical cancers worldwide.[26] HPV invades the body through microscopic cuts in the skin or cervix, [24] so you can catch HPV through intercourse, oral sex or sharing sex toys, even after cleaning (HPV is resilient).[27, 28] Nevertheless, cervical cancer is not inevitable following HPV infection.

HPV infects almost four-fifths (80 per cent) of sexually active women at some time. About 9 in 10 (90 per cent) of these clear HPV during the three years after infection. Only about 1 per cent of chronic HPV infections cause cervical cancer. In addition, most women need to be exposed to other carcinogens – such as smoking, other infections, long-term use of oral contraceptives, AIDS or another immune-related disease – before HPV triggers cancer.[26]

As doctors cannot predict who will develop the cancers linked to HPV, vaccination seems to be a highly effective method of preventing infection. When researchers combined the results from 15 studies including 46,436 patients, they found that:

- vaccination prevented four-fifths (83 per cent) of new HPV 16 and 18 infections over an average of about two years (25.5 months);
- during an average follow-up of 27 months, vaccination prevented 9 in 10 (90 per cent) of chronic (that is, lasting at least six months) HPV 16 and 18 infections;

- when there was an average follow-up of three years (36 months), vaccination prevented four-fifths (84 per cent) of CIN grade 2 or above changes (see page 12).[29]

Nevertheless, screening is important, even if you have been vaccinated. After all, the vaccine does not cover all the types of HPV that potentially cause cancer.

Epstein–Barr virus

Epstein–Barr virus (EBV) is another common virus that seems to increase the risk of certain cancers. EBV belongs to the herpes family of viruses that also includes sexually transmitted herpes and the pathogen that causes chickenpox and shingles. We usually catch EBV during childhood, but EBV is transmitted in saliva, so previously uninfected teenagers commonly catch EBV by kissing.

In adolescents and older people, EBV can cause glandular fever (infectious mononucleosis), with unpleasant symptoms – such as a high temperature, fatigue, a sore throat and swollen lymph nodes in the neck – that usually last 2–3 weeks. EBV remains in the body for life, however, and seems to increase the risk of developing malignancies in the back of the nose and throat (nasopharyngeal cancer), gastric (stomach) and several lymphomas.[2, 30] Worldwide, EBV probably causes about 100,000 cancers a year.[2]

Helicobacter pylori

Fungi and bacteria can also cause certain cancers. For instance, the bacterium *Helicobacter pylori* is remarkably resilient: it manages to survive even in the highly acidic stomach. Indeed, *H. pylori* is probably the most common chronic bacterial infection in humans – more than half the world's population carries the bacterium – and it is the single most common cause of gastric cancer.

Although gastric cancer is the sixteenth most common cancer in the UK – accounting for 1 in 50 (2 per cent) of malignancies – it seems to be the second most common cause of death from cancer worldwide.[2] More commonly, *H. pylori* causes stomach ulcers. A course of antibiotics can eradicate the infection and reduces the risk of stomach cancer by between a third and a half (33 and 44 per cent).

Diet

Cancer is intimately linked to diet, but it is far too large a topic to cover in any detail here. There is plenty of information in books and websites dedicated to the topic, however.

Broadly, eating plenty of fruit and vegetables seems to protect against mouth, throat, oesophageal, stomach, lung and, probably, nasopharynx, colorectal, ovarian, womb, pancreatic and liver malignancies.[31] For example, eating at least seven servings of tomatoes a week seems to reduce the risk of lethal prostate cancer by about a seventh (15 per cent) in men over the age of 60 years.[32]

An unhealthy diet increases the risk of cancer. Rates of prostate cancer are, for example, between half (50 per cent) and three-quarters (75 per cent) lower in vegetarians than those who include meat in their diet.[2] Processed meat seems to be especially harmful:

- if a man with prostate cancer eats 28 g of processed meat a day, his risk of death from the malignancy is a third higher than if he eats none; if he eats 56 g, the risk is a third higher than if he eats 28 g;[33]
- each 100–120 g of red meat eaten a day increases the risk of colorectal cancer by 17–30 per cent;[2]
- each 25–50 g of processed meat a day increases the risk of colorectal cancer by 9–50 per cent.[2]

The fat of the land

An unhealthy diet also increases the risk of being obese or overweight, which appears to increase the risk of developing certain malignancies, including kidney, gallbladder, liver, pancreatic and prostate cancer. Indeed:

- excess body weight caused about 1 in 18 cancers in the UK during 2010 and is the biggest cause of preventable cancer after smoking;[34, 35]
- in women, being overweight and obesity accounted for about 1 in 14 cancers;[23]
- cancer of the endometrium (womb lining) seems to be ten times more common in obese women than among those of a healthy weight;[2]
- a healthy liver contains very little or no fat, but, as your weight increases, fat begins to deposit in the liver; over time, the gradual

accumulation of fat can cause non-alcoholic fatty liver disease (NAFLD); in some people, fat deposits trigger inflammation in and around the liver cells – non-alcoholic steatohepatitis (NASH) – with swelling of, and discomfort or pain around, the liver; over time, NASH can scar the liver; fibrosis (scarring) can progress to cirrhosis, irreversible liver damage and, eventually, liver cancer.[13]

Although patients, professionals and family members worry about cachexia (see page 106) and weight loss, some cancer survivors – such as those on hormonal treatment – gain weight. There is, therefore, a risk that excess weight could increase the risk of second primary cancers. If you want to lose weight, it is best to discuss this with the cancer team once your treatment ends and you have recovered.[36]

Diet during cancer treatment

Eating a healthy diet is *essential* during all three stages of your cancer journey (see page xiii). This is because:

- keeping your strength up and eating a nutritious diet may reduce certain side effects, limit collateral damage and give your treatment the best chance of working;
- during the recovery phase, a healthy diet helps restore your body's well-being and heal any damage from the cancer treatment or the malignancy;
- during the maintenance phase, a healthy diet may prevent or delay a recurrence and reduce the risk of, for instance, second primary cancers, heart attacks, osteoporosis and stroke.[6]

You should see your diet as part of your treatment – as much as the drugs, surgery or radiotherapy. Speak to your cancer team or a dietician, who will be able to offer suggestions tailored to your circumstances and dietary preferences. Note that your cancer team's advice may differ from that for healthy eating generally. For example, in general, everyone should eat a high-fibre diet, but a high-fibre diet could worsen diarrhoea (see page 87) for those receiving certain cancer treatments. Most people need more energy – and so more calories – than usual during cancer treatment. Some drugs also require dietary restrictions to work effectively: certain foods may interact with the medicine, for example.

The cancer team can also refer you to a dietician, who can help with particular issues – such as changes in the way some foods and drinks taste, dry mouth or swallowing difficulties – and support you to make up any nutritional gaps, say with nutrient-rich drinks and other supplements. These range from milk-based shakes to sophisticated, nutritionally complete foods. A dietician can also suggest other modifications to your diet, such as:

- adding butter or cream to certain foods – such as porridge or mashed potato – to increase calories;
- using plenty of gravy and sauces to make swallowing easier;
- taking pre-thickened supplements or adding a 'thickener' to modify the texture of food as this, again, makes food easier to swallow and less likely to 'go down the wrong way', ending up in your lungs.

The cancer team can suggest a range of changes that can help, depending on your particular difficulty. (See also *How to Eat Well When You Have Cancer*, by the specialist cancer dietitian Jane Freeman, listed in Further reading.)

Alcohol and cancer

Heavy drinking increases the risk of more than 200 diseases and conditions, including several cancers. According to the Office for National Statistics (ONS), 29 million people in Great Britain drank alcohol in the week before being interviewed for the 2016 Opinions and Lifestyle Survey. That's about 3 in 5 (57 per cent) of the population. About 3 in 10 men (28.2 per cent) and 1 in 4 women (25.3 per cent) drank more than 8 and 6 units of alcohol respectively on their heaviest day.

Not surprisingly, our national taste for alcohol imposes a heavy clinical load on the already overburdened NHS. According to the ONS, in 2015 there were 8,758 alcohol-related deaths in the UK. Nevertheless, even these sobering figures probably do not paint the whole picture. The ONS estimate includes 'underlying causes of death . . . most directly due to alcohol consumption', such as chronic hepatic disease and liver cirrhosis. The definition excludes, for example, road traffic and other accidents, as well as diseases partly attributable to alcohol, including many cancers.

Indeed, we now know that drinking too much alcohol increases the risk of several malignancies, including cancers in the mouth, throat, voice box (larynx), oesophagus, liver, colon and rectum, pancreas and breast. The risk rises with the amount of alcohol you drink. Even consuming 2.5 units or less a day, however, causes between a quarter (26 per cent) and a third (35 per cent) of deaths from cancer caused by alcohol.[37] That is less than a pint of beer, lager or cider or a 250-ml glass of red or white wine.

The increased risk of cancer linked to alcohol seems to be especially high among smokers. For example, heavy drinking, smoking or both seem to account for about three-quarters of upper aerodigestive tract cancers (malignancies of the lips, mouth, tongue, nose, throat, vocal cords, and parts of the oesophagus and trachea).[38] Alcohol seems to dissolve some carcinogens in smoke, so more of them reach and damage the tissue.

Drinking might also increase the risk of an alcohol-related second primary cancer or the risk of complications following surgery or radiotherapy. For instance, a study of people with upper aerodigestive tract cancers found that:

- continuing to drink after diagnosis increases the risk of complications during and after surgery between two and four times;
- the risk of death due to complications was three times higher in people who, after surgery to remove a tumour, abused alcohol than those who didn't;
- the risk of second primary malignancies was 50 per cent higher in people with upper aerodigestive tract cancers who consumed more than 24 units a week, after allowing for smoking.

Other studies suggest that the increased risk of second primary malignancies might be at least 300 per cent higher for certain upper aerodigestive tract cancers in those who continued to drink.[38]

Furthermore, small amounts of alcohol, even that in certain mouthwashes, might irritate and exacerbate sore mouths (see page 125) caused by some cancer treatments. Alcohol might also interact with some cancer treatments, increasing the risk of side effects. So check with your cancer team whether or not and how much you can drink during treatment and the limits following your diagnosis. Always follow the cancer team's advice: your limit might differ from the government's recommendation.

Cutting back

Some people may use alcohol to help them cope with cancer or its aftermath. If you are going over your cancer team's recommendation or worry you are drinking too much, keep a note of how much you drink – don't just guess. If you drink to alleviate the stress of cancer, speak to your cancer team or GP, who can refer you to NHS Alcohol Services or to a counsellor, who can help you to cut down and deal with difficult situations. Always let the counsellor or support services know that you have or have survived cancer. Some forms of complementary and alternative medicine (CAM) can also help reduce stress that leads to drinking and smoking (see below) and aid relaxation. See also my book *The Holistic Guide for Cancer Survivors* (listed in Further reading) or speak to your cancer team.

How to reduce the amount of alcohol you drink

- Replace large glasses with smaller ones.
- Use a measure at home rather than guess how many units you are pouring.
- Avoid wine with alcohol by volume (ABV) of 14 per cent or 15 per cent. Buy 10 per cent ABV or less.
- Alternate alcoholic and soft drinks.
- Try spritzers and shandies rather than wine and beer.
- Quench your thirst with a soft drink rather than an alcoholic beverage.
- Have several drink-free days each week. You might need to avoid your usual haunts and drinking partners on those days.
- Find a hobby that does not involve drinking.
- Groups buying rounds tend to keep pace with the fastest drinker. Buy your own or buy rounds only in small groups.
- If you rely on a nightcap to get to sleep, try the tips on page 97.

Smoking

Doctors suspected that smoking could cause cancer for centuries. In 1761, for instance, John Hill, a London doctor, reported several cases of nasal cancer among people who used large amounts of snuff.[2] We now know that smoking causes cancers of the lung, mouth, throat, oesophagus, pancreas, stomach, nose and sinuses, voice box, kidney, bladder, uterus, cervix, colon and rectum, ovaries, as well as the blood cancer acute myeloid leukaemia.[2, 39] For example, smoking:

- increases the risk of pancreatic cancer up to three times;[2]
- increases the risk of bladder cancer up to four times and accounts for more than a third of cases of this malignancy in the UK;[2]
- seems to cause 1 in 17 (6 per cent) of leukaemia cases in the UK.[2]

Yet according to government statistics, in 2016, 18 per cent of men and 14 per cent of women in the UK smoked cigarettes.

Even a single cigarette a day increases the risk of cancer. Researchers asked 290,215 adults aged 59–82 years about their cigarette smoking habits and found that:[40]

- deaths from any cause were about two-thirds (64 per cent) higher in those who consistently smoked less than one cigarette a day compared to never smokers;
- consistently smoking between one and ten cigarettes a day increased the risk of death from any cause by nine-tenths (87 per cent);
- people who consistently smoked less than one cigarette a day were more than nine times more likely than never smokers to die from lung cancer;
- people who consistently smoked one to ten cigarettes a day were almost 12 times more likely than never smokers to die from lung cancer;
- people who consistently smoked more than 30 cigarettes a day were about 53 times more likely to die from lung cancer, 25 times more likely to die from respiratory disease and three times more likely to die from cardiovascular disease than never smokers.

It is worth quitting even if you have already developed cancer. A study of people with advanced lung cancer found that continuing to smoke undermined quality of life, for example.[41] Another study found that people who quit smoking after being diagnosed with lung cancer were about seven times more likely to maintain their general well-being and to be able to perform the activities of daily life during the year-long study than those who continued to smoke, even allowing for factors such as treatment and disease stage.[42]

Making quitting easier

- Nicotine replacement therapy (NRT) reduces withdrawal symptoms without exposing you to other harmful chemicals and markedly increases your chance of quitting. Nicotine patches alleviate withdrawal symptoms for 16–24 hours, but begin to work relatively slowly. NRT chewing gum, lozenges, inhalers and nasal sprays act more quickly but do not last as long. Talk to your pharmacist, nurse or GP to find out which is right for you.
- Doctors can prescribe drugs, such as bupropion and varenicline, that help you quit.
- Electronic cigarettes (vaping) contain nicotine, which staves off withdrawal symptoms and means you are not exposed to the chemicals that cause cancer and other diseases linked to tobacco. The wide range of e-cigarettes means you should be able to find one that suits you. However, e-cigarettes can cause mouth and throat irritation. As e-cigarettes are relatively new, any long-term side effects are poorly understood. So use e-cigarettes to stop rather than replace smoking. The risks from second-hand vaping are not fully understood, so limit passive exposure as far as practical.
- Keep a diary of factors and situations that tempt you to light up – such as stress, boredom, a low mood, anxiety and worries, coffee, meals and pubs – then find an alternative. If it is pressure at work or anxiety about the cancer or its treatment that triggers smoking, try stress management, mindfulness or relaxation.
- Hypnosis can increase the chances of quitting smoking almost fivefold.[43]
- Not letting other people smoke in your home helps to strengthen your resolve.
- Try to quit abruptly. People who cut back the number of cigarettes they smoke usually inhale more deeply to get the same amount of nicotine. Reducing smoking takes you a step towards kicking the habit, but do not stop there. Set a quit date as smokers are more likely to quit if they set a specific date rather than saying, for example, that they will give up in the next two months.
- Smoking is expensive. Note how much you save and spend at least some of it on something for yourself.
- Get a free 'quit smoking' pack from the NHS Smokefree National Helpline (0300 123 1044) and contact your local Stop Smoking Service, which offers advice, support and advice about NRT. People who use the service with NRT are up to four times more

likely to quit than those who just try to stop. Speaking to an adviser before your quit date can help you cope with withdrawal symptoms. Always let the adviser know that you are being treated for or have survived cancer.

- Alcohol can sap willpower, so abstinence from drinking seems to improve your chances of quitting. Heavy drinkers are more likely than light or moderate drinkers to continue smoking after being diagnosed with cancer.[38]
- Regard any relapse as a temporary setback. Try to identify why you relapsed. Were you stressed out, anxious or depressed? Did a particular time, place or event cause you to light up? Once you know why you slipped you can develop strategies to stop it happening in future. Then set another quit date and try again.

Genes and cancer

Almost every one of the trillions of cells in your body contains an 'instruction manual' to make your entire body, contained in DNA's famous double helix. The amount of DNA in your body never ceases to amaze me. Pulled into a single, microscopically thin strand, your DNA would go from Earth to the Sun and back more than 300 times, or wrap around the Earth's equator 2.5 million times.[44]

The genes on your 23 chromosomes tell your cells what to do and when: such as when to divide and when to stop. In most cancers, several of the genetic instructions become mutated.

On average, each of us, whether or not we have cancer, has between 40 and 60 genetic abnormalities. Fortunately, few of these mutations cause cancer or another disease. Most mutations do not change the gene's meaning or the body can compensate, so the genetic abnormality does not matter, but some alter the instruction and, in turn, how the cell works.[16]

Biologists have linked around 100 genes to at least one cancer.[45] Some contribute to several cancers and they increase the risk in a number of ways. Some genes lead to cancer when they become inappropriately activated – it is almost as if the mutation presses the cell's accelerator to the floor. Some lead to cancer when they are blocked. These tumour suppressor genes slow cell division: the mutation takes the brake off the cell's division,[17] so the cell divides over and over again.

For example, as mentioned on page 4, p53 is a 'checkpoint' protein that ensures the cell divides properly. The gene that carries the instruction to make p53 is the most commonly mutated gene in cancers generally. Even when the gene that carries the instruction to make p53 is not mutated, other abnormal changes in the pathways leading to or controlled by p53 stop this 'master switch' from working properly.[10] Another gene called *Ras* produces proteins that control the growth, division and differentiation of cells. This critical gene is mutated in about a quarter of all cancers, half of colon cancers and 9 in 10 pancreatic cancers.[10]

Why pancreatic cancers are difficult to treat

Pancreatic cancers are notoriously difficult to treat, partly because an almost impenetrable barrier, called the stroma, surrounds islands of malignant cells. Pancreatic stroma contributes to carcinogenesis, progression, metastasis and drug resistance and suppresses the immune system.[46] Researchers are working on ways to break the barrier down and let drugs reach the malignant cells.

Copying DNA

Cancer-causing mutations can arise in various ways. For instance, when the cell copies the DNA, enzymes 'proofread' the new strands to make sure they carry the same code as the original. Considering our cells divide trillions of times over the course of our lives, they make remarkably few errors. Indeed, for many biologists, it's remarkable that cancer is not even more common than it already is.

The cell has numerous processes to check and repair mistakes in the genetic code, but sometimes these quality control mechanisms miss one – a bit like an editor missing a 'speling' mistake in a book. The gradual accumulation of proofreading errors is one reason why most cancers become more common as we get older.[12] Half of all cancers in the UK are diagnosed in people over 70 years old, according to Cancer Research UK. In addition, we are less able to repair damaged cells as we get older, so age increases the cumulative damage, and, of course, older people have been exposed to carcinogens and unhealthy lifestyles for longer.

In other words, in many cases, whether or not you develop a cancer is simply a matter of luck. Indeed, random DNA-copying errors cause two-thirds of cancers. A sophisticated mathematical model estimated that various environmental factors account for 3 in 10 (29 per cent) of the mutations in 32 types of cancer in the UK. Inherited genes, it estimated, accounted for 1 in 20 (5 per cent) of the mutations, while random copying errors accounted for the remaining 2 in 3 (66 per cent).[47]

However, the importance of the copying errors depends on the malignancy. For instance, copying errors account for almost all (95 per cent) of the mutations in prostate, brain or bone cancers. In a type of pancreatic cancer (ductal adenocarcinoma), DNA-copying errors cause 3 in 4 (77 per cent) of the mutations compared to 1 in 4 (18 per cent) caused by environmental factors and 1 in 20 (5 per cent) due to heredity. In contrast, inherited factors do not seem to be important in lung cancers. DNA-copying errors seem to account for a third (35 per cent) of mutations in lung cancers. Smoking and other environmental carcinogens account for almost two-thirds (65 per cent) of the mutations that drive lung cancer.[47]

Lifestyle factors and inherited genes

Many lifestyle factors linked to cancer – such as smoking and other chemical carcinogens, as well as excessive exposure to sunlight or tanning beds – can mutate genes. Cigarette smoke, for example, contains a chemical called benzopyrene, which binds to and damages DNA. Because of the ongoing DNA damage, continuing to smoke after cancer has been diagnosed can promote the malignancy's growth and metastases.[16]

You inherit mutated genes from your parents. That is why some cancers run in families. For example, *BRCA* genes seem to be involved in pathways that recognize and repair DNA damage.[48] About 1 in 100 women carry a mutated gene – such as *BRCA1* or *BRCA2* – that dramatically increases their risk of developing breast, ovarian and perhaps some other cancers.[12, 48]

- Between half and four-fifths (50–80 per cent) of women with an inherited mutation in *BRCA1* develop breast cancer. This risk is three to five times higher than that in women without these mutations.[17]
- About 2 in 5 (40 per cent) women with *BRAC1* and 1 in 5 or 10 (10–20 per cent) of those carrying *BRAC2* develop ovarian cancer.[2]

Cancers are genetically unstable

Cancers are more genetically unstable than healthy cells, so the longer the cancer survives, the greater the number of mutations they accumulate and the more they differ from their tissue of origin. A cancer probably accumulates six or seven critical mutations between the initial change and metastasis (see Figure 2.1). Each critical mutation marks another step in the cancer's development.

One critical mutation, for example, might result in hyperplasia, another in an early, localized cancer. Another might promote metastasis. Another might mean that the cancer becomes resistant to a particular treatment – a bit like a bacterium becomes a super-bug after evolving resistance to an antibiotic. The cancer continues to divide – and increase in size – between each of these critical mutations.[49]

This genetic instability means that the cancer also accumulates numerous 'passenger mutations'. These mutations do not seem to influence the tumour's progression or the response to treatment. Sorting out which mutations drive the malignancy's growth, which influence the effectiveness of treatment and, in particular, which could lead to new screening techniques and therapeutic targets is one of the most promising and active areas in cancer research.

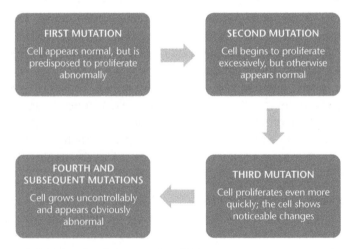

Figure 2.1 Example of the way in which mutations can accumulate in people with cancer

Adapted from M. Bower and J. Waxman, 2015

3

Diagnosing cancer

Diagnosing cancer, especially when the tumour is small enough to be curable, can be difficult. After all, as we have seen, there are some 200 different cancers, each of which can produce a distinctive pattern of symptoms. The average GP in England sees seven new cases of cancer a year.[3] Most of these will be the common malignancies – skin, breast, prostate and so on – so most GPs lack experience recognizing the less common cancers.

Nevertheless, despite advances in screening, about 17 in every 20 cancers are diagnosed after a person presents with symptoms.[1] To complicate diagnosis further, however, many 'minor' illnesses cause the same symptoms as a cancer.[1] Indigestion (heartburn), headaches and backache might be the first sign of gastric (oesophageal or stomach), brain or pancreatic cancer respectively, but they are much more likely to be caused by a poor diet, dehydration and a pulled muscle respectively.

All the same, you should see your GP if the symptom persists. Public Health England, for instance, suggests that people who have indigestion on most days for three weeks or more should see their GP. Always see your GP if you have an alarm symptom or red flag (see Table 3.1). These can also be signs of a recurrence, second primary or progressive cancer.

Unusual symptoms

Sometimes people develop symptoms that are not commonly caused by a malignancy but do turn out to be due to cancer, so it is sensible to get anything unusual checked.

For example, feeling a lump in the breast is often the first indication of breast cancer. In some women, however, the first sign of breast cancer is instead a scab on the breast or nipple that covers a small, weeping sore which does not heal.[10] Indeed, about 1 in 6 women (17 per cent) with breast cancer go to their doctors with

Table 3.1 Examples of alarm symptoms or red flags for cancer[3, 50]

Red flags for lung cancer

Persistent coughing of blood (haemoptysis) in a smoker or an ex-smoker, especially if more than 40 years of age

Breathlessness

Pain in the chest or shoulder or both

One or more of the following symptoms that are unexplained or last for more than three weeks: cough, wheeze or weight loss

---

Red flags for upper gastrointestinal tract cancer (such as stomach and oesophagus)

Dysphagia – difficulty or discomfort swallowing

Persistent vomiting and weight loss

Unexplained iron-deficiency anaemia

Unexplained weight loss

Unexplained abdominal pain and weight loss

A 'mass' (abnormal growth) in the upper abdomen

Jaundice – a yellowing of the skin and 'whites' of the eyes

General red flags

Blood in your stools or urine

Cough that lasts longer than three weeks

Coughing up blood or blood-stained mucus

Diarrhoea that lasts longer than three weeks

Indigestion lasting longer than three weeks or not relieved by medicines, such as antacids

Lump, such as in the breast or testicle, or changes in the way they feel

Rectal bleeding

Swallowing problems (dysphagia)

Unintentional weight loss

---

a symptom other than a lump, according to research presented at the 2016 National Cancer Research Institute conference, such as the following:

- about 1 in 17 women with breast cancer consulted their doctor because of abnormal nipples (7 per cent) or breast pain (6 per cent);
- less commonly, women went to their doctor with back pain (1 per cent) or unexplained weight loss (0.3 per cent);

- other changes that might indicate breast cancer include skin abnormalities, ulcers, changes in shape and an infected or inflamed breast.

Taking a look inside the body

Doctors can look inside your body to see if a tumour might account for your symptoms. For example, they might use ultrasound, X-rays or a flexible camera called an endoscope, which is a thin tube with a camera and light at the end. A surgeon can put the endoscope into your abdomen through a small cut to look at your internal organs on a video screen.

To look in more detail, your team may use computed tomography (CT) or computerized axial tomography (CAT) and magnetic resonance imaging (MRI) scans. CT and MRI scans can visualize the inside of your body in often awe-inspiring detail. Imaging helps diagnose cancer and allows the team to 'stage' the cancer. For example, the cancer team might see if the tumour is restricted to the site of origin, has moved to the lymph nodes or has metastasized.[3]

Plain X-rays and fluoroscopy

'Plain' (standard) X-rays may, for example, detect tumours in the lung or bone, but X-rays often do not adequately differentiate normal and healthy tissue outside the skeleton. So sometimes the radiologist will inject a 'contrast agent', which increases the visibility of some organs and reveals fine detail when using X-rays, CT and fluoroscopy.

The radiologist might also use radioisotopes. These radioactive chemicals accumulate in certain parts of the body where there is increased activity. Some radioisotopes, for example, accumulate where bone is breaking down or being repaired. This helps detect cancers and metastases in the skeleton. Other radioisotopes are absorbed the same way as glucose. Because cancer cells are typically more active than healthy cells, they need more glucose and, in turn, take up more of the radioisotopes.[3]

Fluoroscopy uses continuous X-rays to produce moving images in real time, a bit like taking a video rather than a still image. Fluoroscopy can help surgeons to find obstructions that are blocking the bowel, bile duct or blood vessel, or to image the skeletal, digestive, urinary, respiratory and reproductive systems. The cancer team might also use fluoroscopy to place lines or ports for chemotherapy and to deliver treatment directly to a malignancy, such as microscopic, radioactive spheres to tumours in the liver.[3]

Sounding out cancer

When you are next in a cave or an empty room, shout your name. (Go on – it's fun.) You will hear an echo. The sound wave produced by your voice hits the wall and bounces back. In some caves you will hear more than one echo. The first echoes occur when the sound waves bounce back from nearby surfaces. The more the echo is delayed, the further away is the surface that bounced the sound wave back.

Ultrasound uses a much more sophisticated version of the same general idea. The machine generates high-frequency sound waves that 'bounce back', and create images of the inside of the body. The basic approach used to image cancer is the same as that used to take a scan of an unborn baby. As this suggests, ultrasound is safer than X-rays.

Ultrasound is especially good at assessing malignancies in some organs, such as staging liver cancer. For example, ultrasound can detect liver tumours that are only a few millimetres across. Endoscopic ultrasound inserts the probe into the body on the end of a tube. This is especially valuable for examining the chest – the tube can move along the airways in the lung or down the oesophagus – or abdomen.[3]

Computed tomography

CT uses a beam of X-rays to produce numerous – often more than a hundred – 'slices' through your body, and can image the whole body in a few seconds. The beam varies in width, depending on the level of detail needed. A computer rebuilds the slices into a single three-dimensional, high-definition image. CT is used to stage most cancers, helps plan treatment and evaluate the response, and can detect suspected relapses.[3]

CT delivers a relatively large dose of X-rays, however. According to <www.radiologyinfo.org>, a normal X-ray of your arm – if you have a suspected broken wrist, for instance – delivers about the same amount of radiation you would receive from the normal background sources (see page 14) in three hours. A dental X-ray delivers about the same amount of radiation you would normally receive in a day. A CT scan of the spine or chest, however, delivers the same amount of radiation you would normally receive in two years. A CT scan of the abdomen and pelvis repeated with and without a contrast agent delivers as much radiation as you would normally receive in seven years.

As a result, CT might account for about 1 in 50 (1.5–2 per cent) cancers in the USA.[3] If you are worried about the risks, speak to the cancer team. Cancers typically take many years to develop. Most people with cancer tend to be older or, unfortunately, might have a more limited life expectancy. So even if a scan triggers a cancer, the malignancy might not have time to develop. In other words, the benefits offered by X-rays generally far outweigh the risks.

Magnetic resonance imaging

MRI uses powerful magnetic fields to provide an even more detailed view than CT or ultrasound, so is especially useful when distinguishing healthy and malignant tissue can be difficult (such as in rectal, uterine and cervical cancers). MRI is also often the best way to image the brain and spinal cord to detect cancers and show if a cancer is causing spinal cord compression (see page 11).[3] You must always remind your doctor if you have a pacemaker – MRI might interfere with some pacemakers.[3]

Sampling cancer

Doctors will probably run blood tests and look at a small sample of the tumour or tissue (called a biopsy) under a microscope. During a biopsy the doctor uses a needle to take a small sample of tissue that might be malignant. Usually you will be under a local anaesthetic. In some cases doctors perform the biopsy during an ultrasound or CT scan, which guides the needle to the abnormal area. From the sample, the cancer team can determine whether or not you have a malignancy and ascertain the stage – such as whether the tumour is well- or poorly differentiated (see page 3).

During an operation, the surgeon might take a biopsy of the tissue surrounding the tumour (the margin) or nearby lymph nodes to see if the cancer has spread or to ensure it has all been removed. After surgery the pathologist will examine the tissue removed. This might help characterize the risk of recurrence and assist oncologists in planning adjuvant treatment (see page 39).[3]

During Mohs surgery, commonly used to treat some skin cancers, the pathologist checks the tissue during the operation to ensure all the tumour has been removed. So rather than cut out a lump of tissue, the surgeon takes thin 'peelings'. The pathologist examines the sample during the procedure and tells the surgeon whether or not to take another peeling.[2] Mohs surgery cures almost all primary basal cell carcinomas (99 per cent) and primary squamous cell carcinomas (97 per cent).[2]

Increasingly, medical laboratories test a biopsy to, for example, identify the genetic fingerprint. As we will see later, this can have a big impact on the choice of treatment for some cancers. Indeed, the characteristics and, therefore, the best drug can change over time (see page 68). The cancer team may also examine a sample of your blood for genetic mutations. This allows the team to gain a 'real-time' portrait of the cancer and its response to treatment (liquid biopsy).

Complications of biopsies

Occasionally, biopsies can produce complications, although these are often minor and short-lived. Prostate biopsies, for example, can result in blood in the urine and sperm, difficulty passing urine and erectile dysfunction. For instance:

- between 1 in 17 (6 per cent) and a quarter (25 per cent) of men experience a short-lived exacerbation of urinary symptoms caused by the enlarged prostate;
- just over a third (34 per cent) have difficulty obtaining and maintaining an erection a week after the biopsy (none of the men had erectile dysfunction before the biopsy.)

In general, the complications improve after one to three months.[51] Nevertheless, in one study, 1 in 37 (2.7 per cent) prostate biopsies caused a serious complication, 1 in 86 (1.2 per cent) in hospitalization and 1 in 57 (1.7 per cent) in an infection.[52]

Some parts of the body, such as the liver, have a very rich blood supply. This means that in these parts of the body, a biopsy can cause bleeding. If you have liver cancer, Cancer Research UK warns, there is a small risk that the malignancy could spread along the 'tunnel' left by the needle. The same might apply to some other cancers. Again, have a full discussion with your cancer team – but the benefits usually outweigh any risks.

4

Surgery

Surgery for cancer dates back to at least Ancient Egypt. Despite all the advances in drugs for cancer, radiotherapy and other treatments since then, surgery often remains the best chance for a cure. A surgeon can remove a localized malignancy that has not spread. This depends, of course, on detecting the cancer when the malignant cells remain in one place.

Of course, small cancers are easier to remove than larger tumours. Removing a small cancer is less likely to damage the surrounding area and often produces a better cosmetic outcome than an operation for a larger tumour. Surgery can also:

- prevent some cancers, such as when a surgeon removes pre-malignant tissue;
- repair damage caused by previous operations (such as reconstructive or cosmetic surgery);
- alleviate certain symptoms that might emerge in advanced cancer;
- help treat some recurrences and metastases[2] – indeed, occasionally surgery might cure very limited, localized metastases.[3]

Aims of surgery

Most people with cancer need more than one treatment. Your initial management plan – first-line treatment – might include surgery, chemotherapy and radiotherapy. If the cancer recurs or does not respond adequately, you will move to second-line treatment. If second-line treatment fails, you will move to the third line and so on. The large number of drugs for some cancers means that you could have multiple lines: some women with breast cancer receive 10 or more lines of treatment, for example. In other words, surgery is often one stage in a longer journey.

In many cases, the cancer team will suggest treatment before surgery to shrink the tumour and increase the chance of a good

Thinking about your treatment

Before starting any cancer treatment you should fully discuss the expected risks and benefits with the cancer team. Learning about the treatment can help you understand the importance of sticking to their recommendations and how to deal with and prevent side effects.

You and anyone who might need to help you should think about how the treatment will fit into your lifestyle. You might need to plan childcare, lifts to hospital and work around your chemotherapy sessions, for example. So learn as much as you can about your treatment. The cancer charities are a great place to start to do this, but you should also ask the cancer team some questions, such as the ones listed below.

- Why is this the best treatment for me at this time in my cancer journey?
- What is the goal of treatment? For example, are we trying to cure the cancer or tackle a particular symptom? Is it an attempt to augment the effectiveness of another treatment?
- How and when will I know that the treatment is working?
- How and when will I know that the treatment is not working?
- What are my goals? What do I want to do after the treatment ends?
- How will the treatment help me to reach my goals?
- What are the risks, complications and side effects? How do these compare to other treatments? (You should think about the type and severity of side effects that you are prepared to accept and which would impose an unacceptable burden.)
- Will the treatment affect my quality of life for better or worse?
- What can I do to reduce the risk of side effects?
- Will I need to change my lifestyle or activities?
- What should I do if I miss a dose?
- Whom should I contact if I have any concerns or questions?

You and your family will inevitably have questions, but remembering everything you want to ask in the short time you have in the clinic can be difficult, so keep a notebook or use your mobile phone to jot down any questions. Feel free to make notes and ask questions during the clinic visits. Taking a friend or relative with you might help you understand what you discussed during the visit and can help refresh your memory.

outcome. This could include chemotherapy – for example, for breast or oesophageal cancer – or radiotherapy, such as for rectal cancer.[3]

The cancer team may also use radiotherapy or drugs to mop up any cancer cells that evade the scalpel. For example, using radio-therapy after the operation might allow breast-conserving surgery rather than a mastectomy for a breast cancer.[3] After lumpectomy alone, about half (40–60 per cent) of breast cancers recur. A course of radiotherapy after the surgery reduces the risk of recurrence tenfold (4–6 per cent of breast cancers recur). That is about the same risk as if the surgeon had performed more extensive mastectomy,[2] but the cosmetic outcome is much better. The cancer team works together to plan the best sequence of treatments for you.

Individualizing treatment

Each cancer in each person is unique, so the cancer team individu-alizes the treatment plan depending on several factors, including those listed below.

- **Your general health, well-being and ability to perform the tasks of daily life** The cancer team calls this your performance status. If you are fit and strong, you might be able to tolerate more 'aggressive' treatment that may produce more severe side effects and complications, but offers a better chance of a good outcome, than someone who is more frail.
- **Your goals, plans and attitudes** Some people with metastatic cancer trade a few weeks or months of expected survival for what they see as a better quality of life if that means, for example, they do not experience some side effects. For instance, some men with metastatic prostate cancer are very concerned about losing sexual function, a common side effect of some treatments for this malignancy. As a result, they may refuse surgery or certain drugs that could increase their survival but might compromise sexual function.
- **The site of the secondary tumours and your symptoms** Cer-tain cancers, such as certain primary tumours and metastases in the brain, might be unsuitable for surgery.
- **The treatments – especially drugs – you have received before** Cancers can become resistant to a particular treatment, so a drug

used to treat the primary cancer might not work as well if it or a similar medicine is used to treat metastases.

Ensuring that you receive the right treatment at the right time is one reason why it is so important to have a full and frank discussion with your cancer team before you embark on a course of therapy. You should explore the uncertainties. So if a doctor says you will gain an expected year of life, you might benefit more or less than this. You might not develop the expected side effects or they might be unexpectedly severe. A surgeon cannot guarantee to cure a cancer and will speak instead about 'curative intent'.

The intention of treatment

The intention of treatment might differ depending on the stage of the cancer and your performance status. The cancer team might refer to:[3]

- **radical treatments**, which aim to cure the cancer;
- **palliative treatments**, which aim to control symptoms, extend life or both when a cure is unlikely;
- **neoadjuvant therapies**, which use drugs to reduce the size of the tumour before radiotherapy or surgery;
- **adjuvant therapies**, which use drugs after radiotherapy or surgery to try to mop up any remaining small tumours and circulating cancer cells and radiotherapy can also be used as adjuvant therapy following an operation, as we saw with breast cancer;
- **debulking**, which is when the surgeon removes as much of the cancer as possible, but knows that some malignant cells remain (hence 'debulking'), and the person receives chemotherapy or radiotherapy to remove the rest of the cancer; as such, debulking:
  - increases the chance that the chemotherapy or radiotherapy will kill all the cancer cells;
  - can alleviate symptoms of advanced cancer and increase survival.

Preventative surgery

Some people undergo surgery to remove 'precancerous' lesions, such as small masses of cells called polyps in the stomach or intestine (lesions are areas of cells damaged by disease or injury). Some polyps can develop into gastrointestinal cancer. Similarly, surgeons remove abnormal, precancerous areas of the cervix to prevent cervical cancer.

In addition, some people with a strong family history of thyroid, breast or ovarian cancer might decide to have the potentially affected organ removed.[2] Increasingly, the cancer team can screen to see if you carry the genes responsible for some cancers. For instance, four relatively common genes – *BRCA1*, *BRCA2*, *CHEK2* and *FGFR2* – increase the risk of breast cancer as well as some other malignancies. Four-fifths (80 per cent) of women with one of these genes develop breast cancer, while up to three-fifths (60 per cent) develop ovarian cancer.[2] Some women at high risk decide to have their ovaries or breasts removed to avoid any risk of cancer. Some of these would have never developed the cancer, however, so the operation and the resulting cosmetic and clinical issues were unnecessary. It is a very difficult, very personal decision.

Reconstructive surgery

Often a surgeon aiming to cure a cancer will remove the tumour along with a surrounding 'margin' of healthy tissue and any nearby lymph nodes.[2] This helps ensure that the procedure removes any cancerous cells that have moved into the surrounding area, but surgeons need to strike a careful balance. The more healthy tissue they remove, the greater the potential effect on normal function and, in some cases, the worse the cosmetic appearance.[3]

Reconstructive surgery repairs damage from an operation to remove the cancer or because the malignancy affected a visible part of the body. Advances in cosmetic surgery mean that most people can achieve a good appearance, often despite extensive operations. People with cancer might undergo cosmetic procedures to improve appearance, reduce the psychological burden and enhance quality of life. The best-known example is probably breast reconstruction using, for example, implants, tissue taken from elsewhere in the body or both.[3]

In other cases, reconstructive surgeons might take a flap of skin from, for example, the forearm to repair damage to the face following surgery for head and neck cancer or after an operation to remove a skin cancer in a visible area. The surgeon can replace a lost area of the tongue with a flap of skin, for example. This helps restore speech and swallowing as well as improving the cosmetic appearance. Surgeons can also make tubes from tissue taken from elsewhere in the body, to replace a removed oesophagus (food pipe), for instance.[3]

Helping people with advanced cancer

Surgery can also help alleviate symptoms in advanced cancer. For example, a tumour might block the intestine and, in many cases surgery can relieve the blockage. Surgeons might insert a feeding tube, if you are having difficulty eating, or implant a plastic or metal stent. A stent is a mesh-like tube that can hold open a blocked bowel, food pipe, airway or ureter (carries urine from the kidneys to the bladder).[2]

Surgery can treat some metastases that develop in the skeleton. These secondary bone cancers can cause pain, increase the risk of fractures and hinder normal living.[3] About half of people with metastatic cancer develop a pleural effusion, in which excess fluid accumulates around the lungs. Surgeons can drain the excess fluid.[3]

Before the operation

The operation, associated risks and possible consequences depend on, for example, the cancer, the operation, your particular symptoms and your performance status. So speak to your cancer team and check out the information provided by patient support groups. For example, during surgery for bowel (colorectal) cancer, the surgeon removes the section of the gut containing the tumour, then joins the ends together. In some cases the surgeon passes one end of the gut through the wall of the abdomen to allow the bowel time to heal (a colostomy). The person passes bowel motions into a colostomy bag. Occasionally, the colostomy is permanent.

In breast cancer, the team will discuss the various procedures – such as breast-conserving surgery, mastectomy and reconstruction – to decide which is right for you. In head and neck cancer, a speech and language therapist should discuss the possible effect on speech and swallowing.[3] You might also receive supportive treatments, such as antibiotics to prevent infection or drugs to reduce the risk of venous thromboembolism.[3] If you need major gastrointestinal surgery, you might receive carbohydrate-rich drinks and nutrients that boost the immune system.[3]

You might also take nutritional supplements after the operation, especially if you find you are off your food or have difficulty swallowing. These help your body repair the damage from the operation. Some antioxidants – such as vitamins C and E, zinc, selenium and copper – can improve wound healing, for example.[53]

Venous thromboembolism

In a venous thromboembolism, a blood clot can form in a vein (a blood vessel that carries blood back to the heart). Fragments of this clot can break off, forming an embolism – the word derives from the Greek for throw – that can travel to and block arteries supplying the brain, causing a stroke. Similarly, emboli in an artery supplying the kidney can cause part of this essential organ to die. Emboli in a major vessel supplying the legs can cause gangrene.[54] A fragment that travels to the lungs can cause a blockage called a pulmonary embolism. A large pulmonary embolism can stop the supply of blood to the lung, which can prove fatal.[55]

Reducing the risks of surgery

Advances in surgery have markedly improved the prospects for people with cancer. For example, laparoscopic (keyhole) surgery limits collateral damage to the body. This reduces the need for strong painkillers after the operation, hastens recovery and lowers the risk of complications. Laparoscopic approaches might be appropriate for some breast, colorectal, gynaecological and lung cancers, depending on the size and location of the tumour. Unfortunately, laparoscopic surgery cannot always be used.[3]

Increasingly, surgeons use computer and robotic assistance to further limit collateral damage. For example, during brain surgery, a computer can use imaging data to display the location of the tumour and the instruments as a three-dimensional map on a screen. During robotic surgery, the system can translate the surgeon's movements into smaller, more precise actions at the end of the surgical implement. This allows incredibly delicate procedures, such as removing all or parts of the prostate gland, which is surrounded by a large number of important nerves.[3]

In the early days of breast cancer treatment, surgeons removed all the breast and the underlying tissue, often along with the chest muscle and sometimes even some ribs.[17] Today, surgeons, working as part of the multidisciplinary team, can limit damage to the surrounding tissue while maximizing the outcome. New medicines for cancer often capture the headlines, but advances in surgery have also helped to markedly improve the prospects for people with cancer and helped save countless lives.

5

Radiotherapy

A few months after Röntgen discovered X-rays, Émil Grubbé, a 21-year-old student doctor in Chicago used radiation to treat an elderly woman whose breast cancer had recurred after a mastectomy. After being treated with radiotherapy for 18 days, the cancer had shrunk. Unfortunately, the malignancy metastasized.[17]

Nevertheless, Grubbé's finding suggested that radiotherapy might effectively treat some cancers. Then, in 1899, Thor Stenbeck, a doctor in Stockholm, used X-rays to treat basal cell carcinoma at the tip of a woman's nose. After being treated each day for three months, she became the world's first patient to have cancer cured by radiotherapy.[56]

Since then, X-rays have revolutionized cancer treatment. For example, radiotherapy cures 90 per cent of people with early, low-volume Hodgkin's lymphoma.[2] Radiotherapy can also alleviate symptoms even if the cancer cannot be cured, so, for instance, it significantly reduces discomfort in about half of patients with painful bone metastases, can tackle multiple brain metastases and reduce bleeding caused by some advanced cancers.[3]

Unfortunately, as we have seen, X-rays also cause cancer. Indeed, Grubbé had fingers amputated following radiation damage and eventually underwent 92 operations to treat the consequences of his exposure to high doses of X-rays. He died from multiple metastatic cancers.[17, 57] Moreover, radiotherapy – although it can be lifesaving – may increase the risk of second cancers.

Invisible and painless

Diagnostic radiology uses relatively low-voltage machines to generate X-rays. Therapeutic X-ray machines use a much higher voltage – typically 1,000 times more powerful. This means that the X-rays used to treat a cancer penetrate more deeply and cause more damage than X-rays used to see if you have a broken bone.[2]

Like diagnostic radiology, radiotherapy itself is invisible and pain-less, but side effects are common. You must lie still and follow the radiotherapist's instructions. The radiotherapist will leave the room during treatment to reduce his or her exposure to X-rays.[3] After all, for you the radiotherapy might be a lifesaver, but radiation can also cause cancer and radiotherapists treat several people each day.

Radiotherapy usually fires beams of X-rays at the tumour (external beam radiotherapy). Initially, the radiotherapist will use diagnostic X-rays, CT or MRI (see Chapter 3) to identify the target and see if there are any 'critical' tissues nearby that are especially prone to damage from X-rays. In some cases the radiotherapist might shield healthy tissues (with lead, for example) to prevent damage.[3]

To ensure accurate targeting between radiotherapy sessions, the radiotherapist might make small tattoos on your skin and use bead bags, limb supports and plastic shells to ensure that you do not move during treatment. A plastic mask allows the radiotherapist to deliver the X-rays with millimetre accuracy when, for example, treating a malignancy in the brain or head and neck.[3]

Scheduling radiotherapy

In the early days of radiotherapy, doctors used a single massive dose of radiation, typically lasting an hour. This intense bombardment killed many cells, but also caused considerable damage to healthy tissue.

Radiotherapists now use smaller and shorter doses given over several sessions (fractionated radiotherapy), which are just as effective but much less likely to cause severe side effects. Dose frac-tionation also means that the cancer cells are damaged at different stages in the cell cycle (see page 5).[2]

Between sessions any remaining cancer cells can divide, although usually less rapidly than healthy tissue. Radiotherapy sessions too far apart would allow the malignancy to recover and make the cancer more likely to recur.

Radiotherapy sessions closer together give the cancer cells less time to divide. Some cancers need radiotherapy once a day, up to five days a week for seven weeks. Certain people with lung or head and neck cancer might receive radiotherapy twice a day, but these more intensive regimens also mean that the healthy cells have less time to recover. So more frequent radiotherapy sessions increase the risk of side effects.[3]

Not surprisingly, radiotherapy can be inconvenient. Journeys to the radiotherapy centre can be expensive and take considerable time, which can make it more difficult to perform activities of daily living, including shopping, cooking and eating a healthy diet.[3] You could see if anyone among family and friends can help out. It's important to eat a healthy diet to keep your strength up.

In some cases – for example, certain early breast cancers – you might receive a dose of radiotherapy during the operation. The cancer team might, for example, irradiate the area around the cancer to mop up any small cancers that the surgeons may have missed.

How radiotherapy works

Radiotherapy damages cancer cells by shattering DNA and generating free radicals, which produce breaks in DNA. Cells damaged by X-rays either die immediately or cannot repair themselves and so die more slowly. Radiotherapy often kills cells, inducing necrosis or apoptosis. Even when the cells do not die, cancers repair the damage less effectively than healthy tissue, so the malignant cells are more likely to succumb during the next radiotherapy session.[2]

As cancer cells are less able to repair the damage than healthy cells, radiotherapy tends to damage malignant cells more than healthy tissues. Indeed, radiotherapy can damage cells at any time during the cycle, but affected cells tend to die when the copied chromosomes separate. This means that, depending on how rapidly the cell cycle turns, death of the cell might lag days, weeks or even months after the treatment.[2] Irradiation also damages the blood vessels that supply the tumour with oxygen and nutrients.

Different sensitivity to cancer

Certain cancers are more susceptible to radiotherapy than others (see Table 5.1), so radiotherapy alone might cure highly sensitive cancers. High doses of radiotherapy or lower doses combined with surgery or chemotherapy might cure malignancies that show moderate 'radiosensitivity'. Radiotherapy might only be used as palliation for cancers that show low levels of radiosensitivity.[3]

Free radicals

A slice of apple left exposed to the air soon turns brown. Tissue-damaging chemicals called free radicals cause the colour change. Free radicals are 'waste' products produced by many normal chemical reactions that keep us alive. Our immune system, for example, uses free radicals to help destroy invading bacteria. Free radicals also contribute to the effectiveness of some cancer drugs and radiotherapy.

Free radicals can, however, damage healthy tissue and may increase the risk of certain malignancies, so the body has several lines of natural defence to protect our cells from free radicals – mostly taking the form of a group of chemicals called antioxidants. Unfortunately, pollution, cigarette smoke, pesticides and even sunlight can generate sufficient free radicals to overwhelm these defences. Excessive levels of free radicals seem to increase the risk of developing several serious conditions, including cancers.

Several vitamins, minerals and other antioxidants mop up free radicals, including:

- lutein, found in, for example, green leafy vegetables such as spinach and kale;
- lycopene, the red pigment in tomatoes, apricots, guavas and watermelons (lycopene seems to reduce the risk of developing prostate cancer);
- vitamins A, C, E and selenium.

In general, eating a diet that is rich in antioxidants helps prevent cancer, reduces the risk of a recurrence and boosts your body's innate healing ability. Because free radicals contribute to the benefits of some chemotherapies and radiotherapy, however, your cancer team might suggest avoiding large doses of antioxidants (as supplements, for example) during treatment. Always check with your cancer team.

Combining radiotherapy and other treatments

Chemoradiotherapy – a combination of radiotherapy and chemo-therapy – seems to kill malignant cells more effectively than either used alone, possibly because the chemotherapy makes cancer cells more sensitive to radiation. Chemoradiotherapy can be particularly effective for certain malignancies, especially cervical and oesopha-geal cancers, but can increase the risk of side effects.[3]

Table 5.1 Cancers differ in their sensitivity to radiotherapy[3]

Radiosensitivity	Examples of cancer types
High	Germ cell (see page 53)
	Lymphoma
Moderate	Bladder
	Breast
	Colorectal
	Prostate
	Squamous cell carcinomas of the lung, head and neck, cervix and skin
Low	Kidney (renal)
	Melanoma

For example, a type of hormonal treatment called androgen deprivation therapy (see page 71) combined with radiotherapy improves outcomes in almost all prostate cancers more than either alone. So a man with prostate cancer might receive three or four once-monthly injections with a gonadotropin-releasing hormone (GnRH) analogue (see page 69), which stops once radiotherapy is complete. In high-risk, localized prostate cancer, androgen deprivation might last two to three years, again combined with radiotherapy, but it is worth persisting. In men with prostate cancer, the combination of androgen deprivation and radiotherapy seems to improve survival compared to either alone by about 1 in 10 (10 per cent) over 5–10 years.[3]

Stereotactic radiosurgery

In some cancers – such as tumours in the brain or lung – the cancer team might focus a relatively weak beam of radiation on to the tumour to create a 'hot spot'. The idea is a bit like focusing a sunbeam with a magnifying glass to singe paper. This approach – stereotactic radiosurgery – minimizes damage to the surrounding tissue. Some stereotactic radiosurgery machines use several individual beams focused on the same spot. In other cases, a single beam might be fired at the spot as the radioactive source moves around the head in an arc.[3]

Intensity-modulated radiotherapy

Intensity-modulated radiotherapy often uses eight or more beams to accurately target a tumour. In addition, each beam consists of several 'segments'. Varying the intensity of these segments allows the radiotherapist to build the dose to match the tumour's characteristics and spare healthy tissue. Not surprisingly, planning treatment with intensity-modulated radiotherapy takes longer than does the conventional approach. Intensity-modulated radiotherapy can be remarkably precise, however, sparing the salivary glands when treating head and neck cancer, for example.[3]

Brachytherapy

During brachytherapy, a surgeon or radiotherapist implants small pieces – called pellets or seeds – of radioactive material directly into the tumour, often guided by CT or another imaging technique. The seeds remain in the cancer, destroying the tumour over the next few months as the radioactivity decays to nothing. Another approach inserts a thin tube with a tip containing radioactive material into the cancer. The tube remains in place for several hours or days – depending on the technique – and is then withdrawn.

In brachytherapy, the dose near the radioactive source is very high but falls off rapidly with distance. Indeed, the dose of radiation can fall by 1 in 20 to 1 in 5 (5–20 per cent) per millimetre.[58] This limits the damage to the surrounding normal tissue.[3] Nevertheless, the seeds need to be positioned carefully to ensure that the cancerous cells receive a high dose while limiting exposure of healthy tissue to the radiation. Sometimes the surgeon might implant pellets that deliver a relatively high dose of radioactivity in the centre of the cancer, surrounded by weaker doses to tackle the malignancies in the margins. Brachytherapy can also be used in various combinations with external beam radiotherapy, chemotherapy or both.[58]

Brachytherapy tends to be most effective for tumours that are relatively easy to access, such as cervical and other gynaecological malignancies, prostate cancer and some anal, rectal, breast, head and neck, bladder, skin, liver and eye cancers.[58]

Radioisotopes

As we saw in Chapter 3, some tissues take up and concentrate a radioactive chemical – called a radioisotope or radionuclide – more than others. The thyroid gland concentrates iodine, for example, which it uses to make hormones that influence the way you use energy. Bones concentrate phosphorous, which is used to repair damage to your skeleton. Some thyroid and skeleton will concentrate radioactive iodine and phosphorus respectively.[2] This can aid diagnosis, but at higher doses radioisotopes can also treat some cancers and can, for example, reduce pain caused by metastases in the bone.

Side effects of radiotherapy

Radiotherapy's side effects depend on the dose of radiation, how accurately the technology targets the tumour and the site of the cancer. In general, however, the side effects of radiotherapy include tiredness and weakness, skin reactions and hair loss. The skin reactions caused by radiotherapy range from a faint redness, to sore itchy skin, to weeping and bleeding. Skin reactions tend to peak during the first two weeks after radiotherapy ends and generally resolve within four weeks.[59]

Numerous factors influence the likelihood of developing side effects and their timing, including your ability to repair DNA damage, which part of the body is being treated and how quickly the cells divide.[3] The lining of the mouth (oral mucosa), bone marrow, skin and other rapidly dividing tissues typically develop side effects during or a few weeks after treatment. The early side effects tend to be short-lived. Damage to nerves and blood vessels, which grow slowly, persist long after the end of radiotherapy, however, and might be permanent. Radiotherapy to the chest might, for example, induce heart disease.[3]

Indeed, radiotherapy can cause a wide range of side effects, some of which are listed below.

- Radiotherapy to the brain can cause profound and debilitating fatigue, which might stop you from taking part in the activities of normal life. In addition, radiotherapy to the brain might cause nausea, headache and difficulties with memory and concentration. These effects probably arise because the radiotherapy affects blood vessels and the fatty myelin sheath that surrounds many nerves.[3] The myelin sheath ensures that the nerve signals travel properly.

- Skin reactions usually begin about a week after the start of radiotherapy. The reactions are often worse if the area being treated includes skin folds, such as under the breast or in the groin. Taking chemotherapy and other cancer drugs at the same time might make the reaction worse. The reaction peaks about a week after radiotherapy ends and generally takes two to six weeks to resolve. Long-term skin reactions are uncommon.[3]

- Some people develop inflamed lungs (pneumonitis) between one and three months after radiotherapy, which causes a cough and shortness of breath. In addition, people with pneumonitis may develop a raised temperature, which can make the condition difficult to distinguish from an infection. Usually, pneumonitis does not need treatment. Steroids, which dampen the inflammation, can help severe breathlessness. Smoking can make pneumonitis worse – another good reason to quit.[3]

Long-term consequences

Radiotherapy can induce second primary cancers, which typically emerge at least a decade after treatment ends, although the risk seems to be less than with some types of chemotherapy.

Breast tissue and the thyroid gland seem to be especially sensitive to radiation, which increases the risk of a second cancer (the breast tissue of younger people seems to be particularly sensitive to radiation). People with Hodgkin's lymphoma, however, might need high doses of radiotherapy over a relatively large area of the chest. As a result, women treated with radiotherapy for Hodgkin's disease before reaching the age of 30 years are between 12 and 25 times more likely to develop breast cancer later in life than the general population. The cancer team will probably suggest yearly screening until 50 years of age.[3, 60]

You can also take steps to reduce the risks associated with radiotherapy. For example, among women with breast cancer, smoking seems to negate radiotherapy's benefits and increases the risk of lung cancer and deaths from heart disease (cardiac death). When researchers looked at 75 trials including 40,781 women, those who underwent radiotherapy were twice as likely to develop lung cancer (relative risk 2 in 10) and 30 per cent more likely to die from cardiac causes at least 10 years after treatment than those who did not receive radiotherapy. Using modern treatments, which deliver a lower dose to the lung and heart, the authors estimated that approximately 4 per cent of long-term continuing smokers would develop lung cancer as a result of radiotherapy compared to 0.3 per cent of non-smokers. Approximately 1 per cent of long-term continuing smokers would die from cardiac causes because of radio-therapy compared to 0.3 per cent of non-smokers.[61]

The authors point out that for non-smokers, the absolute risk of death from the side effects of modern radiotherapy is only about 0.5 per cent, which is much less than the benefit. For smokers, however, the risk is about 5 per cent, which is comparable with the benefit. Stopping smoking at the time of radiotherapy will avoid most of the lung cancer and heart disease risk from radiotherapy and has many other benefits.[61] It is best, therefore, to have a full discussion with your radiotherapist or another member of the cancer team.

6

Chemotherapy

Chemotherapy – drugs that, essentially, poison cells – has a poor reputation. Certainly, chemotherapy can cause a range of potentially debilitating and distressing side effects, including hair loss, profound fatigue, as well as nausea and vomiting. Siddhartha Mukherjee notes that cisplatin 'provoked an unremitting nausea, a queasiness of such penetrating force . . . that had rarely been encountered in the history of medicine'. On average, patients in the 1970s taking cisplatin vomited 12 times a day.[17]

Times have, thankfully, changed. Modern anti-emetics can prevent, or at least alleviate, nausea and vomiting for most people. Doctors can choose from a wide range of chemotherapy drugs that allows them to concoct cocktails of medicines that maximize the effect on the cancer, while minimizing side effects. Indeed, although chemotherapy is usually used alongside other approaches in a planned programme of treatment, it can cure a few cancers. For example:

- vincristine helped improve the chances of surviving childhood leukaemia from less than 1 in 10 (10 per cent) in 1960 to more than 9 in 10 (90 per cent) today;
- chemotherapy cures 19 in 20 (95 per cent) of men with testicular cancers that have a good prognosis;
- with chemotherapy, about half (48 per cent) of those with a poor prognosis will still live five years;
- chemotherapy often cures gestational trophoblastic tumours (which derive from the placenta), even in people with widespread metastases, and ovarian germ cell tumours[3] (germ cell tumours begin in reproductive cells: ova in females and sperm in males);
- chemotherapy also cures about half (40–60 per cent) of cases of advanced Hodgkin's lymphoma.[2]

Aims of treatment

Cancers differ in their sensitivity to cytotoxins (cell poisons). Some cancers – such as certain leukaemias, lymphomas, germ cell tumours and childhood malignancies – are highly sensitive, so cytotoxins can cure the malignancy. Other malignancies – such as kidney cancers, melanoma and adult brain tumours – are highly insensitive and chemotherapy is not much use.[2] The sensitivity of most cancers lies somewhere between these extremes.

Usually, therefore, chemotherapy is used alongside other treatments, such as radiotherapy or surgery. Neoadjuvant chemotherapy, for instance, aims to reduce the size of the cancer (called downsizing) to improve the effectiveness of surgery. Neoadjuvant chemotherapy can reduce the size of a breast cancer and avoid the need for a total mastectomy. A less extensive operation might, therefore, remove all the remaining malignancy. In rectal cancer, neoadjuvant treatment might combine chemotherapy and radiotherapy.[3]

Adjuvant chemotherapy follows surgery, to mop up any remaining cancerous cells either locally around the site of the tumour or that have spread elsewhere in the body. Numerous studies show that adjuvant chemotherapy increases survival in a variety of cancers compared to surgery alone. In breast, colon, gastrointestinal, ovarian and lung cancer, for example, adjuvant chemotherapy often begins four to six weeks after surgery. The delay gives the person time to recover from the operation. The course of adjuvant chemotherapy typically lasts three to six months.[3]

Even if the malignancy is incurable, palliative chemotherapy can, in some cases, help improve life expectancy, enhance quality of life and shrink some metastases, which alleviates symptoms in people with advanced cancer. People receiving palliative chemotherapy need to be well enough to tolerate the side effects, however.[3] The balance of risks and benefits is often different if treatment aims to cure a cancer rather than optimize quality of life. Most people would, for example, put up with more severe side effects if there is a reasonable chance of a cure.

This ability to alleviate symptoms is one reason why, despite a reputation for side effects, chemotherapy often improves quality of life. One study, for instance, compared two chemotherapy drugs – docetaxel and mitoxantrone – both given with prednisone (which reduces the risk of allergic side effects), for advanced prostate cancer. In these men, hormone treatments (see Chapter 7) no longer worked. Nevertheless, about 1 in 5 men (22–23 per cent respectively) reported that their quality of life improved with docetaxel compared to 1 in 8 (13 per cent) with mitoxantrone. Docetaxel improved, for example, weight loss, appetite, pain, physical comfort, and bowel and urinary function.[62] Indeed, pain and quality of life can improve rapidly, even after the first cycle (see below) of chemotherapy.

Combination chemotherapy

Essentially, chemotherapy poisons cells. This, in turn, either induces cell death or triggers apoptosis (see page 5).

- Some chemotherapy drugs – such as alkylating agents (platinum compounds, for example) and anthracyclines (such as doxorubicin) – directly damage DNA or RNA (RNA has several roles, including carrying the message encoded in the DNA to the part of the cell that makes proteins). For example, certain alkylating agents and platinum compounds (such as cisplatin) build bridges (called cross-links) between the two strands of DNA or between parts of the same strand. This inhibits the cell's ability to make DNA.
- Other chemotherapy drugs (docetaxel and vincristine, for example) disrupt the cytoskeleton – the cell's scaffolding. This in turn hinders, stops or slows cell division. Spindle proteins, for example, divide the genetic material in a cell equally into two daughter cells (see page 4). Some cytotoxins – such as taxanes (docetaxel, for example) and vinca alkaloids (vincristine, for instance) – stop spindle proteins from working properly.[2, 3]
- Certain chemotherapy drugs (such as 5-flurouracil and capecitabine) interfere with the production of the bases, which are the building blocks of DNA and RNA. Antimetabolites interfere with the pathways that make DNA, protein and RNA.[2]

In other words, chemotherapy drugs stop cell division in a variety of ways. The differences in the mechanisms of action underlie combination treatment, which 'hits' the cancer in two or more vulnerable places. Because the mechanisms of action differ, the patterns of side effects also vary. Doctors might, therefore, be able to combine treatments with side effects that do not overlap, which allows them to administer a higher total dose of chemotherapy.

Imagine, for example, that a drug kills all the cells in a cancer at a dose that causes considerable nausea and vomiting, but does not produce marked fatigue. Imagine that another drug kills the same number of cells through a different mechanism, but at a dose that causes profound fatigue and no nausea or vomiting. If you halve the dose of each and give the person the combination, you will, in theory, kill the same number of cells but markedly reduce the risk of nausea, vomiting and fatigue. You may also experience a wider range of less severe side effects.

Often the cancer team will combine several drugs, depending on the malignancy, the tumour's stage and your ability to tolerate side effects. These combinations maximize the damage to the cancer, limit side effects and reduce the risk that resistance will develop. (As more cancer cells die, there are fewer remaining to develop the genetic changes responsible for resistance.)

For example, up to a fifth (15–20 per cent) of people with leu-kaemia enter remission of the cancer (there was no longer evidence of the malignancy on tests, scans and examinations) treated with methotrexate alone. A similar proportion enter remission after treatment with 6-mercaptopurine. The combination increased the remission rate to almost half (45 per cent).[17] If you have lym-phoma, for example, your oncologist and specialist cancer nurse might discuss combinations with names such as CHOP, VAMP

A metal precious in cancer treatment

In 1965, the American physicist Barnett Rosenberg was studying how electric currents affected a bacterium called *Escherichia coli*. The bacterium stopped dividing, but *E. coli* kept growing, eventually becoming up to 300 times larger than normal, but the electricity also stopped the bacterium from reproducing. Rosenberg used electrodes made from platinum to deliver the electric current. The electrodes produced a chemical called cisplatin, which interfered with DNA replication. Today, cisplatin is used to help treat several malignancies. Indeed, combinations of chemotherapy drugs based around cisplatin mean that testicular cancer, even if metastatic, is usually curable.[2]

(both combinations of four drugs) and BEACOPP (a mixture of seven drugs).

Cycling treatment

You will usually receive several 'cycles' of chemotherapy. You might, for example, receive chemotherapy every day for a few days, followed by a three- or four-week break. This represents one cycle. You then have another few days of chemotherapy, followed by a break. Provided you tolerate the side effects and the cancer responds, you repeat this cycle several times. The timing of the cycles depends on the drug and the cancer's characteristics (such as its sensitivity and how rapidly the cancer divides). Some drugs are more effective as low doses given more often – such as pacli-taxel or cisplatin given weekly rather than a higher dose every few weeks.[3]

In general, the number of cycles depends on the aim of the treat-ment. Adjuvant therapy might, for instance, consist of six cycles. The number of cycles also depends on the sensitivity of the cancer and the cumulative toxicity. So a single cycle might be sufficient as adjuvant therapy for a very sensitive testicular cancer. Palliative treatment of breast cancer with capecitabine usually produces few major side effects and can continue for as long as needed.[3]

Routes of administration

During each cycle, you might receive the chemotherapy in one or more ways:

- as tablets or capsules you take at home;
- by injection or infusion – using a drip or pump – over a few minutes to several hours in hospital;
- administered by specially trained nurses in your home or at a local clinic;
- using a small pump that you wear for a week or more.

In most cases, your choices about the route of administration might be limited, but in some you might be able to discuss the right approach for you. For example, although oral treatment (tablet or capsule, for example) is more convenient, it is not necessarily less toxic than that administered into the bloodstream.[3] You also need to remember to take the oral treatment, which can act as a reminder of the disease (see page 71 for more on remembering to take your medication). If there is a choice, therefore, you and the cancer team need to consider the benefits and disadvantages of the different options carefully.

Sometimes the cancer team might suggest a less common route of administration, such as into the cerebrospinal fluid – intrathecal administration. The cerebrospinal fluid cushions the brain and spinal cord. This means intrathecal administration might be used to, for example, reduce the risk that lymphomas will involve the central nervous system or to treat metastases to the membranes (meninges) surrounding the brain and spinal cord. Intrathecal administration is riskier than an infusion or injection into the bloodstream and the cancer team follows very strict guidelines.[3] Patients with advanced ovarian cancer might receive chemotherapy directly into their abdomen – called intraperitoneal administration.[3]

Tailoring the dose

In general, the effective dose of a drug for a disease other than cancer is considerably less than the dose that causes serious side effects. In other words, the drug has a wide therapeutic window (also called the therapeutic index). Many cancer drugs, however, have a very narrow therapeutic window. The effective dose might even overlap with that which causes serious side effects.

To minimize side effects, the cancer team often needs to calculate the dose carefully. In many cases they will estimate the dose based on your height and weight (strictly speaking, the dose is based on the body surface area, which the cancer team calculates from your height and weight).

In addition, the dose of some cancer drugs depends on how well your kidneys and liver work (renal and hepatic function respectively). Carboplatin, for example, is excreted through the kidneys and the liver breaks down (metabolizes) many drugs. If the kidney or liver do not work as well as they should because of disease or simply age, levels of drugs can accumulate, potentially causing side effects. The cancer team might also change the dose of several other drugs if your kidney or liver become impaired or if you develop certain unacceptable side effects.[3]

Chemotherapy's side effects

Chemotherapy drugs do not discriminate between healthy and cancerous cells: they have the greatest effect on the most rapidly dividing cells irrespective of whether they are malignant or not. Cancer cells generally divide more rapidly than most healthy cells, so chemotherapy tends to have a greater effect on malignant than on most healthy cells. Nevertheless, some healthy cells divide rapidly, which contributes to chemotherapy's side effects. The exact pattern depends on the drug, but the following are typical side effects linked to chemotherapy:

- **nausea and vomiting** chemotherapy damages the rapidly dividing lining of the gut and directly affects the part of the brain that tells us we feel sick;
- **hair loss** follows damage to rapidly dividing cells in the follicles;
- **increased risk of infection** due to damage to rapidly dividing immature white blood cells (see below), which means that you need to be especially careful about hygiene, such as when preparing food, and stay away as much as possible from people with colds and other bugs (your cancer team might suggest taking antibiotics until the white blood cell numbers recover).

As we will see in Chapter 9, you can often help prevent or alleviate many of the common side effects caused by chemotherapy. Your cancer team will offer you advice tailored to the drugs you are receiving and the particular effects they have on you. Ensure that you always know what to do if a side effect develops, rather than wait until it has become established as it can then be more difficult to treat.

Deaths following chemotherapy

All drugs carry risks of potentially serious – even fatal – side effects. Even aspirin can cause bleeding in the gut that, in some people, can prove fatal. Given their potency and their mechanism of action (poisoning cells), it is perhaps not surprising that cancer treatments also occasionally contribute to deaths.

For example, doctors examined 31,183 patients with cancer who were treated in the UK between 2009 and 2013. Of these:

- one in 25 (4 per cent) died within 30 days of receiving chemotherapy, monoclonal antibodies (see page 76) or immunotherapy (see page 79);
- about half (53 per cent) died during their first line of treatment;
- about 1 in 9 of the deaths were definitely or probably related to treatment (6 and 5 per cent respectively);
- certain people seemed especially likely to die within 30 days, including those with a low performance status (see page 38) and other diseases; about 3 in every 5 (56 per cent) of those who died had metastatic cancer.[63]

Infections were the leading cause of the deaths that were definitely or probably related to treatment:

- neutropenic sepsis (see below) accounted for 2 in every 5 deaths (43 per cent);
- pneumonia (11 per cent) and other infections (10 per cent) each caused about 1 in 10 deaths;
- cardiac (heart) problems accounted for 1 in 13 deaths (8 per cent);
- gastrointestinal or vascular (blood vessels) side effects each caused 1 in 50 deaths (2 per cent).[63]

Another study from the UK found that about 1 in 50 (2 per cent) of 271 patients died within 30 days of receiving chemotherapy. The people in the study had a range of solid tumours, including in the breast, lung or prostate.[64]

As ever, it is important to balance these risks against the expected benefits, so have a full and frank discussion with your cancer team. Always ensure you bring any difficulties you are experiencing to the cancer team's attention: only 2 in 5 (39 per cent) of patients who died had contacted their hospital's hotline for advice.[63] It is impossible to say how many lives could have been saved had they called.

Injection site reactions

Many cancer drugs are given by injection or infusion (a slow drip into a vein), which can cause injection site reactions, such as the following:

- some chemotherapy drugs can cause skin blisters or cellulitis (infection of the deeper layers of skin) around the site of infusion (you might need to take antibiotics for these);

- some chemotherapy drugs are irritant, so they can cause red, sore, swollen areas around the needle, as well as discomfort and pain along the vein (your cancer team might suggest non-steroidal anti-inflammatory drugs (NSAIDs) to control the pain and inflammation).[3]

In some cases, the chemotherapy drug leaks into the tissues under the skin (extravasation). The extravasation of some drugs – such as the anthracyclines and vinca alkaloids – can cause pain, swelling, inflammation and discomfort.[3] Sometimes extravasation can damage healthy tissue and, occasionally, might even mean that you lose some mobility in your arm.[3] Always tell your cancer team if you notice changes or experience discomfort in the surrounding tissues after receiving chemotherapy.

Anaemia

Bone marrow produces an astonishing number of new blood cells each day. Production varies from person to person, but, typically, the bone marrow produces, each day, hundreds of billions of blood cells and platelets, which help blood to clot. Given this very rapid turnover, it is not surprising that bone marrow is especially sensitive to the effects of chemotherapy – a side effect called myelosuppression. Colony-stimulating factors – also called haematopoietic growth factors – increase production of blood cells. As such, colony-stimulating factors support people who receive cancer treatments that reduce production of blood cells in the bone marrow.

Some people develop anaemia from low levels of iron, either through blood loss or because their diet suffers.[3] For instance, changes in the way some foods and drinks taste (see page 107) can mean that some people with cancer cannot face red meat, which is a rich source of iron.

Myelosuppression can also cause anaemia. Red blood cells carry oxygen around the body, so low levels of red blood cells can cause unpleasant symptoms, including tiredness and lack of energy, shortness of breath, a pale complexion and heart palpitations.

Your kidneys naturally produce erythropoietin, which triggers red blood cell production. For example, when you visit a mountainous part of the world, your body needs to acclimatize to the lower levels of oxygen, so at higher altitudes your kidneys pump out more erythropoietin, which increases the amount of red blood cells your marrow produces.

Your cancer team might suggest treatment with erythropoietin, which increases red blood cell production and, in turn, might alleviate tiredness, breathlessness or weakness caused by anaemia. Erythropoietin's effectiveness varies widely, however, increasing red blood cell counts by between a fifth and almost two-thirds (20–60 per cent). Up to almost a third (30 per cent) of people with cancer need a blood transfusion to treat anaemia.[2]

Neutropenia

Chemotherapy can reduce the production of white blood cells (leucopoenia), which help fight infections, bacteria, viruses and fungi. One type of white blood cell – neutrophils – accounts for about half of all white blood cells.[8] Unfortunately, neutrophils seem to be especially susceptible to chemotherapy, and levels of this important white blood cell can fall dramatically. This leaves the person very vulnerable to bacterial infections.

Treatment with granulocyte colony-stimulating factor (G-CSF) increases levels of white blood cells and so reduces the risk of infections.[16] For example, white blood cell counts typically decline to their lowest level seven to ten days after chemotherapy. Levels then recover, reaching normal counts after about 21 days. So a typical schedule might be one treatment with chemotherapy every three weeks. By boosting levels of white blood cells, G-CSF can allow chemotherapy to be given once every two weeks, which may improve its effectiveness.[3]

Febrile neutropenia – a high temperature in a person with a low neutrophil count – is the most common cause of treatment-related hospital admissions in cancer patients. As febrile neutropenia is potentially serious, it needs to be recognized and treated rapidly with antibiotics, which have helped to dramatically reduce deaths. If febrile neutropenia is not treated, sepsis can develop, characterized by a dangerous drop in blood pressure and a rapid heart rate.

Neutropenic sepsis can be fatal, so you should immediately tell a member of your cancer team if you develop a temperature over 38 °C (98.6 °F). Nevertheless, as infections in people with neutropenia do not always cause a fever, you should also tell your cancer team if you develop other hallmarks of infection, such as a sore throat or cough.[3]

Thrombocytopenia

Bone marrow makes platelets, which account for between 1 in 20 and 1 in 10 (5–10 per cent) of the cells in your blood.[8] When you cut yourself, for example, the damaged blood vessels send out 'distress signals'. Platelets rush to the cut and form a plug (clot) to stop the bleeding and help the wound heal. Chemotherapy can reduce levels of platelets, which doctors call thrombocytopenia.

Typically, thrombocytopenia causes bruising and bleeding without marked trauma or injury. A purplish rash might be another sign. Often people with thrombocytopenia find that their gums and nose ooze blood. (A heavy flow of blood is not typical of thrombocytopenia, however.)[3] See your cancer team of GP if you develop any of these symptoms.

Bone marrow transplants

To help tackle myelosuppression (see above), you might receive a bone marrow transplant. Allogeneic transplants come from a donor. Alternatively, the cancer team might take bone marrow or harvest stem cells from you before you receive chemotherapy. Stem cells can develop into any blood cell. They replace the marrow or the stem cells once you have received treatment (autologous transplant). The stem cells then divide repeatedly and repopulate the bone marrow.[2]

Bone marrow transplants can allow you to receive much higher doses of chemotherapy than you could otherwise: often myelosuppression is the first 'major' (dose-limiting) side effect to emerge. If you do not develop myelosuppression or receive a bone marrow transplant, the cancer team may be able to at least double the dose before the next dose-limiting side effect (often mucosal damage – see page 108) develops. Bone marrow transplants have limitations, however, including a risk of death, so it is important to fully understand the risks and benefits.[2]

Tumour lysis syndrome

Occasionally the damage to some cancers – especially to certain lymphomas and leukaemias – causes the 'tumour lysis syndrome'. These cancers are highly sensitive to chemotherapy and the damage releases a flood of chemicals, including those that were part of the DNA, into the blood. The risk is especially high at the start of chemotherapy, when the cells are most sensitive. The high levels of chemicals can cause potentially dangerous disturbances to the heart rhythm or damage the kidneys. Indeed, some people might need urgent dialysis. Most people who develop the tumour lysis syndrome, however, have a potentially curable cancer.[2] Again, discuss the potential risks and benefits with the cancer team.

Lung injury

Lung symptoms often arise in people with cancer when the disease progresses – such as from lung metastases – or they pick up a lung infection. Doctors are, however, increasingly aware that some chemotherapy regimens can directly damage the lungs, producing symptoms that emerge weeks, months and occasionally years after chemotherapy ends.[3]

Researchers still need to work out many of the details, but it seems that the drugs cause inflammation and scarring in the lungs. Although lung injury sometimes proves difficult to manage, the cancer team can offer a range of treatments that may help, so see your doctor if you develop breathlessness, malaise, fatigue or a non-productive cough (that is, one that does not bring up mucus).[3]

Heart damage

Some chemotherapy drugs can damage and inflame muscles in the heart. Over time this can cause increasing fatigue, fast heart rate, pulmonary oedema (fluid in the lung) and congestive heart failure. Indeed, women treated with anthracyclines (epirubicin and doxorubicin) for breast cancer are half as much again (50 per cent) more likely to die from heart disease than those who received other chemotherapies. Again, these symptoms might not emerge until many years after chemotherapy ends.[3]

Men treated for testicular cancer are also more likely to develop cardiovascular disease, partly because of the side effects with cisplatin and partly because of low levels of hormones. This makes them more likely to show risk factors for cardiovascular disease, such as dangerously raised blood pressure (hypertension), changes in cholesterol and other lipids, and obesity. Many of these risk factors can be managed with, for example, drugs to lower blood pressure and cholesterol levels, a healthy diet and regular exercise.[3]

Heart failure

Heart failure arises when the heart 'fails' to pump enough blood to meet your body's demands. Doctors divide heart failure into two types.

- **Left heart failure** The heart cannot pump enough of the blood that it receives from the lungs. Blood backs up in the lungs (pulmonary oedema), causing breathlessness.
- **Right heart failure** The heart cannot pump enough of the blood received from the body. Blood backs up in the legs, ankles, torso and so on, leading to puffiness of the hands, feet or face, discomfort and skin ulcers. The 'congestion' is why doctors often refer to this as congestive heart failure.

Second primary cancers

As mentioned above, some cancer drugs directly damage DNA. This means that the cancer drugs may increase the risk of a second primary cancer, which often emerges several years after the treatment of the first malignancy ends.

Some chemotherapy drugs can, for example, induce acute myelogenous leukaemia. The risk begins to increase one to two years after treatment with alkylating agents, peaks after five to ten years and then declines. Unfortunately, these leukaemias often prove difficult to treat. The overall risk depends on the drug, the combination, the total dose and the duration of therapy.[60]

Leukaemia patients are about six times more likely to develop a second primary cancer than the general population. Lymphoma survivors are about five times more likely to develop a second primary cancer. Young people seem to be especially vulnerable to the effects of chemotherapy. Patients diagnosed with leukaemia or lymphoma at 10 years of age or younger are about 11 times more likely to develop a second primary cancer than the general population. Adults are about four times more likely to develop a second primary cancer.[3] It is important, therefore, to follow an anti-cancer lifestyle to reduce your risk of developing second primary cancers. Your cancer team, patient group or my book *The Holistic Guide for Cancer Survivors* (listed in Further reading) offer further advice.

7

Hormonal treatment

Hormones are chemical messengers released by glands around the body – such as the pituitary, pineal, thyroid, testicles, ovaries and pancreas. The thyroid gland produces thyroid hormone, for instance. The testes produce testosterone, while the ovaries secrete oestrogen. Hormones are essential for our health and well-being, controlling, for example:

- metabolism, including the conversion of food into energy;
- some aspects of mood and emotions;
- reproduction and sexual function;
- growth and development.

Some cancers are especially sensitive to hormones' growth-promoting effects. Oestrogen, for example, drives many cases of breast cancer, and testosterone often stimulates prostate cancer. So drugs that block these hormones are important treatments for breast, prostate and some other 'hormone-sensitive' (also called 'hormone-dependent') cancers.

Receptors and cancer

Hormones act by binding with specific 'receptors' on their target cells (see Figure 7.1). Imagine a cell is a car. The receptor is the ignition; the hormone is the key. When the key is slotted into the ignition, the engine can start and the car move. Similarly, when the hormone binds to the receptor, part of the cell's internal machine starts and the cancer grows. This binding is specific: your key starts only your car; testosterone does not bind to oestrogen receptors, for example. Many of the body's other messengers – such as the neurotransmitters that pass signals between nerves and from nerves to muscle – also act by binding to receptors.

Imagine you have a skeleton key that fits the ignition and switches on the engine. Some drugs act like a skeleton key. That is,

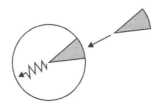

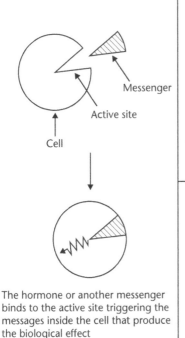

Agonists bind to the active site and trigger the messages, producing the same biological effect as the messenger or hormone

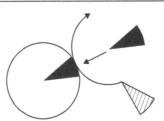

The hormone or another messenger binds to the active site triggering the messages inside the cell that produce the biological effect

Antagonists bind to the active site and don't trigger the messages, but they prevent the messenger from binding, so blocking the biological effect

Figure 7.1 Drugs, hormones and receptors

the receptor cannot distinguish the drug (called an agonist) from the messenger produced by the body; both switch on the cell's machinery. For example, your brain produces natural painkillers called endorphins (also known as endogenous opioids) that bind to specific receptors. Morphine, commonly used to treat severe cancer-related pain, binds to the same receptors as the endorphins and switches on the same pain-relieving pathways.

Imagine that you have another key. It fits the ignition, but will not turn, so the car will not start. While this key is in the lock, however, you cannot get the right key in. Some drugs operate in a similar way, binding to the receptor but not activating the cell's machinery. These are antagonists. About 7 in every 10 breast cancers express oestrogen receptors. Drugs that block the oestrogen receptor are important treatments for early and advanced breast cancer.[3] Anti-androgens (such as bicalutamide, cyproterone acetate and flutamide) attach to testosterone receptors, stopping the hormone from stimulating prostate cancer.

Receptor status

Because receptors are specific, a drug that interferes with hormones will work only if the cancer is sensitive to that hormone, so the cancer team will test a sample of the malignancy to see if it expresses receptors for the hormone. For example, oestrogen and progesterone stimulate the growth of some breast cancers, so the team will test for receptors for these two hormones and classify the malignancy as:

- oestrogen receptor positive (ER+) or negative (ER-);
- progesterone receptor positive (PR+) or negative (PR-).

Doctors call this the cancer's 'receptor status'.

As mentioned earlier, cancers are genetically very unstable and can change as they develop, so a primary breast cancer that is ER+ can produce ER- metastases and vice versa. One study found that the receptor status for breast cancer metastases differed from the primary malignancy in about 1 in 6 cancers (18 per cent) for oestrogen and almost half (45 per cent) for progesterone.[65] The cancer's receptor status can influence treatment, so it is worth discussing taking a biopsy of breast cancer metastases with your cancer team. Not all metastases can be sampled, however, as they might be inaccessible, for example.

Blocking hormones

Blocking the hormone that stimulates the malignancy's growth or preventing its production can help treat hormone-sensitive cancers. For instance, many women with ER+ breast cancer take tamoxifen, which blocks oestrogen. Tamoxifen locks on to the oestrogen receptors. This means that oestrogen cannot stimulate the cancer cells' growth and division. Tamoxifen can control advanced breast cancer, although resistance usually develops, and lowers the risk of early breast cancer coming back (recurring) after surgery or developing in the other breast. One study followed women with early breast cancer for 15 years. Over this time, taking tamoxifen for five years reduced the risk of death from breast cancer from a third (33 per cent) to a quarter (24 per cent). Taking tamoxifen for five years also reduced the risk of recurrence from about half (46 per cent) to a third (33 per cent).[3]

Most prostate cancers depend on testosterone to grow. Luteinizing hormone (LH) controls production of oestrogen and progesterone by the ovaries and testosterone by the testes (see below). Doctors might suggest drugs that block LH for some prostate and breast cancers. As mentioned previously (see pages 5 and 55), essentially chemotherapy works by directly killing cells or triggering apoptosis. Drugs that block hormones typically work at another stage in the cell cycle: they reduce cell proliferation.[3]

As we shall see in the next chapter, hormonal treatments might be combined with targeted treatments, such as trastuzumab (Herceptin), lapatinib (Tyverb) or everolimus (Afinitor).[3] The combination allows the treatment to 'attack' the cancer on more than one front. Hormonal treatments can also help control some more advanced cancers, such as small visceral and bone metastases from breast cancer.[3]

The choice of hormonal treatment depends on your malignancy and other factors. For example, ovaries stop making oestrogen after the menopause, so LH blockers work for breast cancer in premenopausal women only. If the cancer no longer responds to a hormonal treatment, doctors describe it as 'hormone refractory'.

Prostate cancer

In healthy men, an area of the brain called the hypothalamus releases gonadotropin-releasing hormone (GnRH). The hypothalamus is just above the pituitary gland, which lies behind the bridge of your nose. The pituitary controls the action of many other glands. The pulses of GnRH trigger the pituitary to release pulses of LH and follicle-stimulating hormone (FSH).

LH stimulates testosterone production in the testes, while testosterone and FSH trigger sperm production. Testosterone from the testes is released into the circulation and feeds back to the hypothalamus and pituitary gland, reducing production of GnRH, FSH and LH.[66, 67]

A group of drugs called GnRH analogues disrupt this 'feedback' loop[3] ('analogue' means it is similar in shape to GnRH and so binds to the same receptor). GnRH analogues trick the body into acting as if levels of testosterone are high, so after an initial rise (flare), levels of testosterone fall dramatically. The flare can stimulate the tumour, which might lead to difficulty passing water and, in some people, result in spinal cord compression. As a result, the cancer team will probably prescribe a drug that blocks testosterone's effect on the tumour and other tissues for two weeks before giving the GnRH analogue. You generally receive a GnRH analogue as an injection into the fat under your skin every month or once every three months.[3]

Aromatase inhibitors

Aromatase inhibitors are the main hormonal treatment for breast cancer in post-menopausal women. In addition to the ovaries, an enzyme in fat (called aromatase) makes oestrogen. Aromatase inhibitors lower oestrogen levels by blocking this enzyme. Aromatase inhibitors do not, however, stop the ovaries from producing oestrogen. The aromatase inhibitors, therefore, only lower oestrogen levels in women whose ovaries are not producing the hormone, such as those who have been through the menopause.

Side effects of hormone treatments

Hormones control some very basic aspects of our biology; after all, you cannot get much more basic than reproduction. For example, testosterone increases muscle strength, so blocking testosterone might trigger fatigue and weakness. (Men produce low levels of oestrogen, just as women produce low levels of testosterone.)

While side effects are common, in most people the benefits of hormone treatments outweigh the risks. In many cases some simple steps can help alleviate the discomfort – have a full and frank discussion with your cancer team.

During the natural menopause, for example, oestrogen levels fall. This means that drugs which block oestrogen can cause symptoms similar to the menopause, but, unlike the natural menopause, these symptoms can arise in men. About 7 in 10 women undergoing hormonal treatment for breast cancer and a similar proportion of men taking some drugs for prostate cancer experience hot flushes.

Tamoxifen, for example, might cause hot flushes, vaginal dryness, loss of libido and weight gain.[3] In rare cases, tamoxifen seems to increase the risk of endometrial cancer and disorders of blood clotting (thromboembolic disease), so always tell your cancer team if you develop abnormal bleeding, such as from the vagina or gums. As tamoxifen affects blood clotting, you might stop treatment before an operation. In premenopausal women, tamoxifen can also weaken bones, leaving you more vulnerable to fractures.[3]

You can take steps to manage some of these side effects (see page 113). For example, taking drugs such as tamoxifen in the evening might reduce hot flushes (but never change your dose schedule without speaking to your cancer team first). Your cancer team can also suggest a variety of drugs that might alleviate hot flushes. Some people find hypnosis, acupuncture and yoga reduce flushes. A lubricant may alleviate vaginal dryness. Painkillers, weight loss, exercise and physiotherapy can reduce joint pain.[3]

In men with prostate cancer, GnRH analogues can cause hot flushes, impotence and weight gain. Some drugs can cause breast tenderness and growth in men (gynaecomastia) or damage your liver. Long-term treatment might weaken bones. Prostate cancer seems to increase the risk of diseases affecting the heart and blood vessels (cardiovascular system). Androgen deprivation appears to further increase the risk. So your cancer team might suggest treatments to protect your bones and cardiovascular system.[3]

Aromatase inhibitors can cause joint and muscle pains, loss of libido and weaken bones. Taking vitamin D and calcium supplements, and drugs that strengthen the skeleton (bisphosphonates), can help minimize the effect on bones. You might also need bone scans to monitor the effect on your skeleton.[3] Other side effects are specific to each treatment, so speak to your cancer team and check out the information provided by cancer charities (see Useful addresses).

Remembering to take your treatment

Remembering to take your treatment can be challenging, especially if you have several drugs to remember (including for ailments other than the cancer), you feel depressed and demotivated or the drugs or cancer affect your memory (see the box 'Cancer-related cognitive impairment'). Here are some ideas you might like to try.

- Ask your partner or carer to remind you to take your medicine.
- Keep a checklist and cross or tick each dose when you take it. Some apps track your medicine use. If you share this either electronically or by pinning up the list, your partner or carer only needs to remind you if you have forgotten.
- Leave yourself notes reminding you to take your treatment on the refrigerator, over your desk, next to the television, on the bathroom mirror, wherever works for you.
- Leave your medicines where they are easily seen, such as on the dining or bedside table or desk. Always keep medicines out of reach of young children, however.
- Speak to your cancer team if you have difficulties opening the packaging or swallowing tablets – there are often ways around these. If you have joint pain, for example, a pharmacist can repackage the medicines in containers that are easier to open. Liquid formulations of some medicines can help if you have difficulty swallowing.
- Try to take your treatment at the same times each day, which helps establish a routine and, in turn, helps you remember. You could use an alarm on a watch, phone or timer to remind you.
- Your routine might change on holiday, on a day out, at a birthday, wedding or if you are away on business. You might need to adjust your timings. Make sure you have sufficient supplies of all your medicines while away. Remember that you might not be allowed to take some painkillers into certain countries, so always check.

Some people feel that alarms are intrusive and remind them they are ill. If the alarm goes off in public, you might not want to explain about your cancer. You might feel irritated if carers remind you to take a medicine when you already have. Everybody is different, so find what works for you.

Intentionally refusing treatment

The practical steps given above can help if the person with cancer unintentionally forgets to take his or her medication, but sometimes people intentionally don't take their medicine as suggested. Indeed, in one study, more than half (55 per cent) of those taking

Cancer-related cognitive impairment

Some people with cancer find that it is hard to concentrate, focus or pay attention, which can linger after the initial treatment ends. Some report memory loss or difficulty remembering names, dates or phone numbers or with comprehension or understanding. Numerous factors linked to cancer and its treatment can cause or worsen cognitive impairment, including some chemotherapy drugs, hormonal therapy, certain forms of radiotherapy, stress, chemical changes produced by the cancer and brain tumours. Up to 3 in every 10 patients experience cancer-related cognitive impairment before chemotherapy. This rises to up to three-quarters during treatment – so-called 'chemo-brain' or 'chemo-fog'. The symptom persists for several months after treatment for more than a third (35 per cent) of patients.[68]

drugs – including tamoxifen – for breast cancer did not take their medicine as recommended, frequently or occasionally. About 4 in every 5 (83 per cent) of those who did not take their medicines said they forgot, but about 1 in 6 (17 per cent) reported that they intentionally did not take their medication.[69]

Some people deliberately did not take their medication to avoid side effects, such as hot flushes. If side effects make you reluctant to follow the suggested regimen for taking your medicines, speak to the cancer team. Often there is a lot they can do to help.

Other people who deliberately missed their medication viewed themselves as having significantly less influence over their health and well-being than those who followed their cancer team's advice.[69] Perhaps some people feel that not taking a treatment helps re-establish a sense of control. Others might not fully appreciate the benefits of treatment, especially if they experience cancer-related cognitive impairment.

Obviously, a cancer treatment will not work unless you take it. So, if you are deliberately not taking your medicines, speak to your cancer team and explore the reasons underlying your reluctance. Ultimately, the choice is yours. During palliative care or in advanced cancer, for example, you might refuse a treatment or trade a less effective approach for one with fewer side effects. Nevertheless, self-help tips and, if necessary, supportive treatments can often manage side effects, so do not suffer in silence. If you feel you are not in control, try complementary or alternative medicine (CAM) or counselling instead of ignoring your team's advice.

If you are caring for someone with cancer and you suspect he or she is not taking the medicines as suggested, you should gently and non-judgementally raise the issue with the person or the cancer team. You could save or prolong that person's life.

8

Targeted treatments and immunotherapy

As mentioned previously, researchers now have an unprecedented understanding of cancer biology – although we are still a very long way from fully understanding malignancies. Nevertheless, these insights have resulted in a new generation of high-profile medicines that have transformed the prospects for certain cancers: the targeted treatments and immunotherapy. The mechanisms through which these drugs produce their biological effects can be difficult to understand, even for healthcare professionals. After all, some of these mechanisms are at the cutting edge of biological science and, in some cases, many of the details have not been worked out fully. Check out the information for patients on charities' websites (see Useful addresses) and do not be afraid to ask questions.

Targeted treatments

Targeted treatments (sometimes called biological therapies) influence specific processes that control cancer cells' growth, division, spread and death. So, for example, a messenger might bind to a receptor (see page 66) on the surface of a cancer cell. This binding triggers a chemical cascade inside the cell that transmits the signal from the receptor to the nucleus of the cell. The nucleus contains the cell's DNA and other parts of its genetic machine; the signal tells the machinery to 'switch on' the genes that drive an aspect of the cancer's growth.

You could block this pathway at several stages. You could stop the drug from binding to the receptor, so the messenger cannot trigger the message – some hormonal treatments and certain targeted treatments work in this way. You could block one or more steps in the cascade inside the cell – certain targeted treatments work in this way. You could damage the DNA and stop the cell from dividing – as chemotherapy drugs do.

Most targeted treatments aim at receptors or stages in the pathway that are unique to, or very much more active in, malignant than healthy cells, and drive the cancer's growth and development.[3] This limits side effects, although scientists have yet to develop a magic bullet that targets cancer and leaves healthy tissue untouched.

Unfortunately, targeted treatments are often expensive, which has led to several high-profile cases in which the NHS claims that it cannot afford to fund cancer drugs to gain a few months' extra life or reduce the risk of adverse events.

Antibodies

Some types of white blood cells produce antibodies, which identify and help remove invading viruses, bacteria and other pathogens. Antibodies 'stick' to the microbe or infected cell, which allows the immune system to home in on the pathogen or damaged cell. Antibodies mean that we mount a much more rapid immune reaction next time we encounter the same invader, which is why vaccines protect us from some serious diseases.

Many targeted treatments are artificially created 'monoclonal antibodies'. These allow the cancer team to hit a very specific target, such as one protein from among the many thousands produced by a cell. (That is one reason why researchers distinguish passenger mutations from those driving the cancer's growth and development: see page 28.) For example, trastuzumab (also called Herceptin) and bevacizumab (also called Avastin) are both monoclonal antibodies, although, as we will see, they have very different targets.

Blocking growth factors

Some targeted therapies – such as trastuzumab, gefitinib and imatinib – block growth factors. As the term 'growth factors' suggests, these messengers tell cancers to grow and spread. For example, receptors called HER2 bind a messenger called 'human epidermal growth factor'. Between 1 in 7 and 1 in 4 breast cancers express very high numbers of HER2 receptors (HER2-positive malignancies). These malignancies tend to grow more quickly than HER2-negative breast cancers. Some gastric (stomach) cancers also express high levels of HER2 receptors. If you have one of these cancers, the cancer team will test a sample of tissue to ascertain your HER2 status.

Trastuzumab binds to HER2, which stops the receptor working properly. This interrupts the growth factor's signal. You will receive trastuzumab only if you are HER2 positive. In about 1 in 7 (13 per cent) of patients, HER2-positive primary breast cancer can produce metastases that are HER2 negative and vice versa [65] – another reason to discuss taking a biopsy of any secondary tumours (see page 68).

Blocking blood vessels

Other targeted therapies – including bevacizumab – block the formation of the new blood vessels that supply the growing tumour with oxygen and nutrients. Very small tumours can absorb oxygen and nutrients from the fluid that bathes each cell, but a tumour larger than about one-tenth of a millimetre needs its own blood supply.[16] So the cancer releases chemicals that stimulate the growth of new blood vessels – a process called angiogenesis. Some cancer drugs block the messengers that control angiogenesis. This starves the cancer of oxygen and nutrients. Bevacizumab, used to treat a range of cancers, targets a messenger that drives angiogenesis called vascular endothelial growth factor.

Different patterns of side effects

Targeted treatments are much more specific than traditional chemotherapy, so they cause less collateral damage. The side effects differ from treatment to treatment, but, in general, diarrhoea and skin rashes seem to be the most common side effects triggered by biological and targeted treatments.

The immune system evolved to identify and attack proteins that are not made by the body. The antibodies used to treat cancer are 'foreign' proteins. Unfortunately, the immune system does not distinguish between a medicine and a pathogen. Although the antibodies are developed to reduce the risk of a reaction (by being as close to natural human antibodies as possible, for instance), the immune system might still recognize that these are foreign and mount an attack. In some cases this attack triggers an allergic reaction; in others the body might produce antibodies against the targeted treatment – and the levels of these 'neutralizing antibodies' can sometimes be high enough to stop the drug from working.

Certain side effects reflect the mechanism of action, such as increased bleeding with drugs that target angiogenesis.[3] You should always discuss possible side effects with the cancer team and know what to do if you think they have emerged. If you are in any doubt, always seek medical attention.

The immune system and cancer

Your immune system protects you from viruses, bacteria and fungi as well as destroying abnormal, damaged and cancerous cells. Many CAMs seem to stimulate the body's innate healing abilities, including boosting the immune system. Indeed, occasionally the body's innate response is strong enough to lead to the complete or partial disappearance of a malignancy when the patient is not receiving a conventional treatment that could explain the improvement. Doctors call this a 'spontaneous remission'.

Spontaneous remissions

A 44-year-old woman underwent surgery to remove a tumour in her left breast. Some 11 years later, a scan detected another lump in the same breast. A biopsy showed that the cancer had returned and her surgeons planned another operation. A month after the biopsy, however – and before she underwent surgery – the woman noticed that the lump was smaller. Ultrasound the day before the planned operation confirmed that the cancer had regressed. Indeed, a biopsy found no cancer cells in the mass. Most of the lump seemed to be scar tissue. It seems that the cancer had vanished.[70]

Spontaneous remissions are more common than many patients – and probably cancer teams – realize, and seem to occur for almost every type of cancer.[71] Nevertheless, many doctors seem unwilling to 'recognize, appreciate, and investigate' spontaneous remissions.[72] As a result, 'massive under-reporting' hinders attempts to work out how often spontaneous remissions occur, though there have been some studies of this phenomenon. A Japanese study of 311 breast cancers from 308 patients found that 1 in 14 (7 per cent) of the tumours regressed spontaneously. The average cancer was 2.8 cm across and all the tumours that regressed were highly malignant.[73] Other studies suggest that between 1 in every 100,000 and more than 1 in 10,000 cancers might spontaneously enter remission.[72]

Some spontaneous remissions last for years. For example, spontaneous remissions in renal cell carcinoma (a malignancy in the kidney) have lasted between 3 months and 20 years. Nevertheless, most patients relapse eventually[71] and a spontaneous regression is only rarely a cure. Metastatic cancer is generally incurable, however, and in many advanced cancers, even the most effective modern treatment usually only buys time.

Spontaneous remissions probably account for the case histories of remarkable cures used by some CAM practitioners. Interestingly, about two-thirds of patients experienced 'some kind of spiritual awakening' before the spontaneous remission, suggesting that they had 'a central role in the process of healing'.[72] Indeed, in many cases, the mind seems to stimulate an immune response that attacks the cancer. It is less clear, however, why this immune response only occurs in some people. Nevertheless, the recognition of the immune system's importance in our natural defences against cancer has led researchers to suggest that it might offer a new approach to treatment – so-called immunotherapy.

Immunotherapy

Immunotherapy, which leverages the immune system's power to tackle cancer, is one of the most active and promising areas in cancer research – it has been standing room only when some results have been presented at scientific conferences. The lay press heralded immunotherapy as 'effectively' curing some terminal cancers.[74] Also, at the time of writing, about half of cancer clinical trials include a variant of immunotherapy.[75, 76]

I'm old enough to recall, however, the 'global media hype' that surrounded interferon, claiming it would be 'a "magic bullet" against cancer' in the late 1970s and early 1980s. The body releases interferons (a group of proteins that pass messages between cells) to boost the response to viruses, bacteria, parasites and cancer cells. So, used as a drug, researchers hoped that interferon would activate the immune system and boost the body's ability to destroy malignant cells.[76]

In large cancer studies, however, interferon was disappointing. In some cases, interferons can overstimulate the immune response more generally, producing, for example, flu-like symptoms, rashes or swelling around the injection site, and fatigue. Many patients experienced severe side effects. Eventually, interferons found several niches, but they are a long way from being the possible cures for cancer the headlines suggested.[76, 77] So, should we believe the hype this time?

An old idea

The basic idea underlying immunotherapy is not new. Physicians in the 1700s noted that some malignancies improved when patients contracted bacterial infections. In the late nineteenth and early twentieth centuries, physicians attempted to induce immune responses to control cancer. For instance, in 1893 a New York surgeon called William Coley used a bacterial vaccine to induce a strong immune response in people with inoperable cancers. Coley reported some impressive results for the time, such as a cure rate of better than 10 per cent for inoperable sarcomas.[2, 76, 78]

More recently, scientists found that some tumours containing large amounts of white blood cells show a better prognosis than those which do not.[2] (Some white blood cells destroy cancerous cells.) Indeed, researchers have long realized that the immune system can eliminate cells during their initial transformation into cancer – called immune surveillance.[79]

The failure of immune surveillance helps account for the increased risk of some cancers in certain people with suppressed immune systems, such as those with AIDS or who are taking drugs to reduce the risk of rejecting a transplanted organ.[2] For example, Hodgkin's lymphoma (a cancer of the lymph nodes) is ten times more common in people with HIV and two to four times more common in people who receive an organ transplant.

- People with organ transplants are at increased risk of several malignancies, including Kaposi's sarcoma, non-melanoma skin cancer and cervical cancer. Heart and heart–lung transplants require the most potent immunosuppression, so the risk is greater than with kidney transplants.[2]
- In people with HIV, Kaposi's sarcoma, non-Hodgkin's lymphoma and cervical cancer are the most common malignancies.[2]

Indeed, several conventional cancer chemotherapies stimulate the immune system. Some rearrange the proteins that the immune cells use as a target (called an antigen) on tumour cells. This allows the immune system to 'detect' the cancer. Others undermine the mechanisms that the tumour uses to evade the immune surveillance. Others directly or indirectly stimulate immune cells.[80] So it is clear that the immune system is important in driving cancer, but it was many years before drugs that specifically aimed to attack cancer by affecting the immune system became clinical reality.

The many faces of immunotherapy

There are several types of immunotherapy that are either being used to treat cancer or investigated in clinical studies. Each type of immunotherapy works through a different mechanism. Some of these, at the time of writing, are still being developed – you can keep up to date with the latest advances by checking out the patient group websites.

Vaccinating against cancer

First, doctors increasingly *treat* cancers with a vaccine. Vaccines protect against serious diseases by enhancing your immune defences. When you are exposed to a virus or bacteria, a vaccine-boosted immune system can usually eradicate the infection before symptoms develop, so, as mentioned previously (see page 15), some vaccines prevent cancer. The vaccine against human papilloma virus (HPV), for example, boosts your defences against this virus, which can cause cervical cancer and some head and neck malignancies. People with chronic hepatitis B virus (HBV) are up to 100 times more likely to develop hepatocellular carcinoma (the most common liver cancer) than the general population. Indeed, the vaccine against HBV was the first immunization that prevented a specific human cancer.[14]

Therapeutic vaccines treat certain malignancies by stimulating an immune response to the cancer.[79] In some cases, doctors use samples of the cancer to develop vaccines against the tumour. These vaccines will be specific to your cancer. Other 'non-individualized' vaccines target a specific protein expressed by the cancer but not healthy tissue. In both cases, the vaccine stimulates the body's white blood cells to attack and, hopefully, destroy the malignancy.

Unfortunately, many tumours 'hide' from the immune system – so-called tolerance. Overcoming tolerance depends on identifying and expressing a target that the cancer produces in large amounts, but is not produced by healthy tissue. These cancer-specific antigens allow the immune system to target the malignancy and influence survival or growth. Identifying the most suitable antigens often proves difficult, however.[79]

Viral attack

The second approach uses viruses that replicate in and kill cancer cells and not healthy tissue. These 'oncolytic viruses' reduce the size of the tumour and the damage to the tumour triggers the body's immune system to attack the cancer. The damage to the tumour, for example, can release the cancer's antigens, which triggers the immune attack. Genetically engineered oncolytic viruses can also work as biological factories, pumping out chemical messengers that stimulate immune reactions. To evade the immune system, oncolytic viruses tend to be injected near the malignancy. However, this means that they might not reach metastases and some tumours might be inaccessible to injection.[79]

Using your white blood cells

During another approach – called adoptive cell therapy – the cancer team isolates lymphocytes (a type of white blood cell) from the patient's blood, lymph nodes close to the cancer or the tumour. The number of lymphocytes is increased in the laboratory, after which they are reinfused back into the patient. In some cases, these transplants induce dramatic and durable responses. For example, between half and three-quarters (49 to 72 per cent) of melanomas respond. In about 1 in 5 (22 per cent) patients, the cancer completely disappears. Growing the lymphocytes in the laboratory takes time and is relatively costly, however. At the time of writing, further studies are needed to characterize the long-term benefits and side effects.[79]

Antibodies versus checkpoints

The final group of immunotherapies block the checkpoints in the pathways that inhibit the immune response against the cancer (see page 4). Essentially, the approach 'reawakens' the immune cells inside the cancer.[75] For instance, pembrolizumab targets a checkpoint protein called PD-L1 (programmed death-ligand 1). In one study, researchers used pembrolizumab to treat non-small cell lung cancer (NSCLC) that progressed after the patients had received standard chemotherapy. About 1 in 5 people (19 per cent) showed a response and average overall survival was 12 months. Another study reported that about two-fifths (44 per cent) of patients with previously untreated brain metastases caused by NSCLC responded.[81] As we have seen (see page 11), brain metastases can prove particularly difficult to treat.

These are only examples. Other immunotherapies targeting one of several checkpoint proteins are showing promising results in a variety of cancers. The side effects depend on the drug and, at the time of writing, further studies are needed to clarify the risks and benefits. We already know, however, that some checkpoint inhibitors, for example, can cause adverse events when activated immune cells infiltrate healthy tissue, such as the gastrointestinal tract, lung, liver and pituitary gland.[81]

Further studies are needed – we are only beginning to scratch the surface of this promising approach – so stay up to date by looking at the cancer charities' websites. Immunotherapy does not work for everyone, but it might, for example, find an important role as an adjunct therapy to mop up circulating cancer cells left by the primary treatment.[76] Immunotherapy seems set to become a mainstay of management for many malignancies, alongside radiotherapy, chemotherapy and surgery.

9

Coping with side effects

This chapter offers some tips that might help prevent or manage particular side effects. Given the wide range of cancers and treatments, and because individual susceptibility varies from person to person, these are only general tips. *Any advice that your cancer team offers overrides these suggestions.* If you feel unwell at any time, contact your GP or cancer team. Many of these tips are also covered in my book *The Holistic Guide for Cancer Survivors*, which places a greater emphasis on the role of CAMs in combination with conventional medicine.

Nausea and vomiting

Nausea and vomiting are among the most feared and distressing side effects of chemotherapy and certain malignancies. Unfortunately, they are also relatively common: between 1 in 10 and 1 in 4 people receiving chemotherapy endures persistent nausea and vomiting, for example.[82] Furthermore, at least 7 in every 10 people with advanced cancer report chronic nausea.[83] Some cancers cause nausea and vomiting by, for example, affecting the gastrointestinal tract or changing the blood's chemistry.

The likelihood of developing nausea and vomiting depends on the drug and the patient. Cisplatin and mustine, for instance, commonly cause vomiting. Vinca alkaloids, in contrast, rarely trigger nausea. Certain people – such as women, younger people and those who have been sick previously with chemotherapy – are at especially high risk of developing nausea and vomiting.[2]

Interestingly, the more you expect – based on what you have heard or on previous experience – to develop nausea and vomiting when you receive chemotherapy, the more likely the symptoms are to occur.[82] Nausea and vomiting – which evolved to expel hazardous material before it can do you harm – are among our body's strongest and most basic reactions. Occasionally, even the thought or a reminder ('cues') of the chemotherapy is enough to trigger the reaction – so-called anticipatory nausea and vomiting. Doxorubicin, for instance, is a red-coloured infusion that commonly causes nausea and vomiting. Some patients, therefore, experience nausea and vomiting when they see the colour red outside the chemotherapy suite.[82] Counselling and hypnosis can help break any psychological link between anticipatory cues and nausea and vomiting.

Anti-emetics

Anti-emetics are drugs that reduce the frequency and severity of nausea and vomiting. Your cancer team might suggest that you take anti-emetics – which include ondansetron, granisetron and aprepitant – before and for 24–48 hours after chemotherapy. You might receive additional treatment if you develop 'breakthrough' nausea and vomiting during chemotherapy or 'late' nausea and vomiting, which is when it occurs 3–5 days following chemotherapy.[3] Radiotherapy can also cause vomiting in the minutes or hours after treatment begins. Again, anti-emetics can help reduce the frequency and severity of the nausea and vomiting.[3]

Self-help tips for nausea and vomiting

The self-help tips listed below might also help to prevent nausea and vomiting.[3, 82, 84, 85]

- Avoid fatty, greasy and fried foods. Eat small amounts of plain foods when you feel able, such as:
  - baked, boiled or mashed potatoes rather than chips;
  - turkey or chicken, with plain noodles or rice, instead of red meat;
  - poached egg on dry toast.
- Grape juice might reduce the frequency and duration of nausea and vomiting.
- If the smell of cooking triggers nausea, eat cold meals or prepared foods.
- Dry foods, such as toast and crackers, might help settle a sensitive stomach. Some people find that dry foods work best if eaten in the morning.
- For centuries, traditional healers have used ginger to alleviate nausea from a variety of causes. Try crystallized ginger, ginger tea or ginger biscuits.

- Vomiting can lead rapidly to dehydration, so sip plenty of drinks – such as ginger beer, mineral water, lemonade or soda water – slowly through a straw. If you find a straw difficult to use, try a bottle with a sports cap.
- Rinse your mouth before and after meals, which helps get rid of any lingering tastes.
- Sit up or lie back with your head raised for at least an hour after eating rather than lie down.
- Relaxation techniques – such as meditation and mindfulness – can help reduce nausea and vomiting before eating.

Constipation

Several factors can trigger constipation in people with cancer, including some painkillers, certain drugs used to treat nausea and vomiting, dehydration and several malignancies.[3] If you think you have constipation, record how many times you pass a bowel movement and the consistency. Ideally, use the Bristol Stool Chart, which is widely used by doctors and nurses (<www.hct.nhs.uk/media/1067/bristol-stool-chart.pdf >) to describe this. Do not take laxatives – even those bought without a prescription – unless your cancer team tells you to. Seek medical advice if the constipation is severe or painful or you are worried.

Self-help tips for constipation

The tips listed below might help you prevent or alleviate constipation.[3]

- Dehydration can make stools harder, so drink between six and ten glasses of fluid a day. This can include water, prune and other fruit juices, lemon squash, fizzy drinks and soup. Some people find that not drinking alcohol, coffee, tea and grapefruit juices, which can make you urinate more, helps prevent dehydration.
- Take regular exercise, ideally for at least 30 minutes a day.
- Try to have regular bowel movements. You might find defecating after breakfast easier than at other times as this is when the bowel's contractions tend to be strongest. Try to go to the toilet at the same time each day, which helps establish a routine.

- Eat more fibre. Good sources include:
  - porridge or a wheat biscuit cereal;
  - peas, beans and lentils – you can add these to a soup or stew;
  - stewed or tinned fruit; mashed banana;
  - vegetables – again, you can add these to stews, soups and casseroles.

Diarrhoea

Diarrhoea in a person with cancer can have numerous causes, including:

- the cancer you have;
- certain treatments for cancer or other diseases;
- infections;
- irritable bowel disease;
- excessive use of laxatives;
- reducing the dose of or stopping some painkillers, such as morphine and other opioids;
- stress and anxiety.

If you think you have diarrhoea, keep a check using the Bristol Stool Chart (see 'Constipation' above) and note any triggers. Doing this often helps identify the cause. If you have four or more episodes a day, see your doctor as soon as you can.[3]

Usually diarrhoea triggered by chemotherapy is mild and manageable with lifestyle changes and antidiarrhoeal drugs. Occasionally, however, diarrhoea is more serious. Indeed, the chemotherapy drug irinotecan can cause severe, even life-threatening diarrhoea.[3] Always tell your cancer team if you experience severe diarrhoea. You should also contact your doctor urgently if you develop a fever and abdominal pain alongside the diarrhoea. This might indicate a potentially serious infection of the wall of the large bowel.[3]

People undergoing radiotherapy might find that they pass stools more often, the stools might be softer and there might be colicky pain or wind. This can develop into diarrhoea, which can be accompanied by mucus ('slime') or small amounts of blood.[3] Again, ask your cancer team what to expect and speak to them if you are worried.

Self-help tips for diarrhoea

Sometimes doctors might prescribe – or advise you to buy – anti-diarrhoeal drugs, such as loperamide. They may suggest you keep this at home and start taking the drug at the first sign of diarrhoea. Otherwise, however, never buy or use a treatment for diarrhoea – or any other symptom – without speaking to your cancer team first: some antidiarrhoeal drugs could cause additional difficulties or interact with other elements of your treatment.

The tips listed below might help alleviate diarrhoea without the need to take something for it. [3, 85–87]

- Avoid high-fibre, fatty, greasy and spicy foods. Try eating plain food – such as bananas, white bread, white fish, chicken or turkey – in small, frequent meals.
- Eat foods rich in pectin, which is the natural gelling agent found in ripe fruit used to make jams and jellies. Eating less fibre and more pectin-rich foods helps build stool consistency (see Table 9.1).
- Diarrhoea may mean that you lose large amounts of a mineral called potassium, which nerves and muscles, for instance, need to work properly. Losing large amounts of potassium can leave you feeling weak and fatigued. Eating foods high in potassium helps replenish your stores of this vital mineral (see Table 9.1).
- Diarrhoea can lead rapidly to dehydration, so drink at least 2–3 litres a day, including water, lemon squash, fizzy or still drinks

Table 9.1 Foods rich in pectin, potassium or both

Foods rich in pectin	Foods rich in potassium
Apple, peeled or as sauce, without spices	Apricot nectar
Asparagus tips	Asparagus tips
Avocados	Avocados
Banana	Bananas
Beetroot	Fish
Plain pasta	Peach nectar
Potatoes, baked, without skin	Potatoes, boiled or mashed, without skin
White bread	
White rice	

and clear soups or drinks made from beef stock cubes or extract. Some people find that avoiding caffeine, alcohol, fruit juices and smoothies helps alleviate diarrhoea, but make sure you get enough fluid in other ways.

- Probiotics help restore the natural balance of bacteria in your gut, which can become disrupted by cancer and its treatment as well as by supportive care, such as antibiotics. Changes to the balance of bacteria in the gut can trigger diarrhoea. Ask your cancer team or dietician if you are not sure which probiotic is right for you.
- Try eating foods at room temperature: cold and hot foods tend to stimulate the gut.
- Good hygiene is very important if you develop diarrhoea. Clean yourself carefully after each bowel movement. Use soft wipes and pat rather than rub. You can apply a barrier cream to protect the delicate area around the anus. Ask your cancer team or a pharmacist if you are not sure which barrier cream to use.

Bladder symptoms

Some people with cancer experience difficulties urinating, either because of a cancer or its treatment. Radiotherapy, for example, can damage the bladder, causing symptoms that include pain on passing urine, increased frequency and blood in the urine. In general, bladder symptoms emerge during or soon after radiotherapy, but they might emerge up to a year after treatment ends. Your cancer team will rule out infections, which can also cause bladder symptoms.[3]

If you develop bladder symptoms, ensure that you drink sufficient fluids. Some people find taking cranberry capsules helps.[3] If these do not improve the symptoms, your cancer team can prescribe several drugs that might restore bladder control.

Fatigue

Fatigue is one of the most disabling and distressing symptoms experienced by people with cancer. People with cancer-related fatigue feel tired all the time and physically, emotionally and mentally exhausted. Rest and sleep do not alleviate their profound tiredness.

Preventing dehydration

Anyone, whether or not they have cancer, can easily become dehydrated as they go about their daily lives. Even in healthy people, the mild dehydration that might arise during our daily activities can cause a range of symptoms, including:[88, 89]

- constipation
- poor concentration and memory
- increased tension or anxiety
- fatigue
- headache.

Some people with cancer have additional issues that make dehydration more likely. You might experience difficulties swallowing, for example. You might feel too fatigued to get yourself a drink. You might lose fluids because of diarrhoea or vomiting. Whatever the cause, everyone should stay hydrated.

The NHS suggests that adults should drink 1.2 litres (six to eight glasses of water) each day to replace fluids lost in urine, sweat and so on. This is, however, an average: personally, I need to drink more than this. (Excessive thirst and increased urination might be a sign of diabetes, however, so see your GP if you experience these symptoms.) If you feel thirsty for long periods, you are not drinking enough. You should drink more during exercise, hot weather or when you are in a warm ward or chemotherapy suite. You should also drink more if you feel lightheaded, pass dark-coloured urine or have not passed urine for six hours.

Self-help tips for bladder symptoms

The tips listed below might help you to ensure you get enough fluids.

- Carry a water bottle with you and take sips throughout the day. Some nutritional supplements are sipped between meals, which can also help keep you hydrated. Ask your cancer team to speak to a dietician if you think this will help.
- If you are too fatigued to get up regularly, make sure you keep plenty of bottles of water by your chair or bed.
- Choose recipes with plenty of gravy, sauces, custards and cream. Keeping food moist can also help you if you have difficulties swallowing.

- Try different drinks – such as malted milk drinks or beef extracts, milk shakes, soups – provided these do not dull your appetite for meals. These can also boost your intake of protein, energy and other nutrients if eating enough food at mealtimes is difficult.
- Although you need to drink regularly, try not to consume too much during meals. Fluids can make you feel full up sooner and blunt your appetite.
- If you have lost fluids due to vomiting or diarrhoea, try a drink with electrolytes, such as ones developed for use after a workout. A pharmacist or your cancer team can suggest electrolyte drinks.

The body, especially arms and legs, might feel heavy. People might experience difficulty concentrating or cannot think clearly. Indeed, some people with severe cancer-related fatigue might be unable to perform everyday activities, such as eating, shopping, working, exercising or even personal hygiene.[12]

Unfortunately, such symptoms are common. At least four-fifths (80 per cent) of people with cancer experience fatigue during chemo- or radiotherapy, and most (60–90 per cent) regard fatigue as their most disabling symptom.[83] Occasionally fatigue is so profound that patients discontinue treatments, contemplate suicide or wish for an early death.[83] So how can you reduce fatigue's impact?

Causes of cancer-related fatigue

There are numerous causes or contributors to cancer-related fatigue.[12, 83, 87, 90]

- Fatigue can emerge as your body recovers from surgery or as a side effect of chemo- or radiotherapy.
- Some cancers release chemical messengers that undermine your energy. When chemo- and radiotherapy destroy the cancer, the tumour might release a flood of chemicals into the blood that triggers sleep difficulties and fatigue.
- Disrupted sleep, anaemia, infections and poor nutrition can all cause or exacerbate fatigue.
- Cognitive symptoms, depression and pain can make fatigue worse. Depression, for example, can sap your motivation and energy. In turn, fatigue can increase the likelihood of cognitive symptoms, depression and pain. It is all too easy to become trapped in a

downward spiral. Once again, speak to your cancer team if you feel any of these issues could be making matters worse.

Doctors sometimes inappropriately blame psychological factors when their suggestions fail to alleviate cancer-related fatigue. Keep a diary of your symptoms. This can help you and your cancer team to identify the causes of fatigue and the impact on your ability to perform the normal activities of daily living and on your quality of life. Understanding the triggers and consequences helps identify the best ways to help you. You should record:[84]

- **how bad the fatigue feels** try ranking its severity on a scale of '0' for no fatigue or tiredness to '10' for the worst fatigue you have experienced or can imagine;
- **how much the fatigue interferes with your daily life** you could rank this from '0' for no interference to '10' for being unable to get out of bed or out of a chair;
- **your sleep patterns** this helps reveal any link between your fatigue and, for example, poor sleep hygiene or poorly controlled pain;
- **your daily activities** this helps identify any triggers in your lifestyle, such as trying to do too much or having too many visitors;
- **what you have tried to address the fatigue and any improvement** you could rate how well strategies have worked on a scale of '0' for no improvement to '10' if the fatigue resolved.

Self-help tips for cancer-related fatigue

Unlike nausea, vomiting and pain, few drugs can help people with cancer-related fatigue, unless anaemia, an infection or depression contributes.[87] Fatigue often improves after the cancer treatment ends and is worst early in the journey. It seems that as people learn to live with the cancer, they know what to expect – the severity of cancer-related fatigue sometimes comes as a shock – and what helps. This means that you need to take a proactive approach to dealing with fatigue.

Planning, prioritizing and pacing

Planning, prioritizing and pacing allow you to spend your time and energy on those activities that you value most or need to get done.[83, 85, 87, 91]

- List things that you *have* to do and what you can leave or ask someone else to do.
- List the most important things for you – the things you really *want* to do.
- Jot down who you can ask for help, for what and when (so that, for example, it fits into their commitments). Family and friends are usually more than willing to help, but often do not know what to do or feel uncomfortable asking. They could help by, for example, giving you a lift to hospital, looking after children, cooking or with the housework. Often your family and friends will feel better because they can do something.
- Your diary can help you strike the right balance between rest and activity. Plan your daily routine, which should include regular rest and relaxation. You might find that you need to add extra periods of rest before or after activity or visitors. Take a break if you feel you need to rest, even if it is unscheduled. Struggling on just makes matters worse. Nevertheless, excessive rest can sap your energy and interfere with sleep, so work out the ideal amount for you.

Find time to exercise

You might not always feel up to a workout, especially if you are fatigued, your muscles or joints ache or you feel depressed, yet regular exercise brings important benefits for people with cancer.[12, 36, 68, 83, 84, 92]

- Physical activity is, ironically, one of the best ways to counter fatigue. That is one reason why regular exercise helps you look after yourself and improves your quality of life.
- Many people find that exercise alleviates anxiety, depression and stress.
- Exercise might reduce the impact on your body composition of the cancer and its treatment. Exercise, for example, strengthens muscles and bones, and improves heart and lung function.
- Exercise can help counter nausea and vomiting, sharpen your appetite, improve digestion and prevent constipation.
- Exercise might help prevent and alleviate lymphoedema (see page 111), 'menopausal' symptoms linked to hormonal treatments, and cancer-related cognitive impairment.

- Exercise might improve survival. For instance, women with breast cancer who reduced their physical activity after their malignancy was diagnosed were twice as likely to die in the next eleven years than those who maintained or increased their exercise levels.[93]

Speak to your cancer team before beginning exercise or physical activity. You might need to adapt your diet or you might be vulnerable to certain injuries. For example, people with skeletal metastasis or bone loss due to therapy should avoid activities that could increase the risk of fractures, such as jumping or twisting the hips. Chemotherapy-induced neuropathy might affect balance, which means you should exercise in a way that avoids the risk of falls.[36]

Some other tips for living with cancer-related fatigue

Here are a few more tips that might help you live with cancer-related fatigue.[83, 85, 87, 91]

- A motorized scooter might help preserve your independence.
- You could ask your cancer team or GP to refer you to an occupational therapist, who might be able to suggest changes that could be made to your home that could help conserve energy, such as grab rails, raising toilet seats or putting chairs near stairs.
- Overuse of painkillers, sedatives and some other drugs can cause or contribute to fatigue. If you suspect that a treatment could be a factor, speak to your cancer team. There is a usually an alternative. Never stop a treatment or reduce the dose, however, unless advised to do so by your cancer team.
- Some people find that fatigue undermines their memory and concentration. Try making notes, keep lists and stick to a routine.
- Try to distract yourself. Watch a DVD, read or listen to music or a podcast – anything that takes your mind off the cancer and your fatigue.
- Try to take part in activities you enjoy several times a week.
- After checking with your cancer team, try a CAM, such as yoga, mindfulness, meditation, guided imagery or progressive muscle relaxation.
- Think about your diet. Cells use a sugar called glucose as fuel. Digestion breaks complex carbohydrates into glucose more slowly than it breaks down simple sugars (such as the sugar in your

tea), so you might find that eating, for instance, rice, chapattis, yams, noodles, cereals, pasta, potatoes and bread maintains your energy levels better than filling up on simple sugars.

Fatigue experienced by carers

Carers often endure profound tiredness and marked sleep disturbances. After all, caring for someone with cancer can be mentally, physically and emotionally exhausting. Carers:

- might need to prioritize demands on their time and plan accordingly;
- might benefit from stress and time-management techniques;
- should try to get enough rest and relaxation;
- should take part in activities they enjoy at least a couple of times a week;
- discuss respite care with the cancer team and the person with cancer – recharging your batteries will help improve the care you are able to give to the person with cancer.

Sleep disturbances

Disturbed sleep in a person with cancer can have numerous causes, including that it is a:

- symptom of the cancer;
- side effect of several medications;
- result of poorly controlled pain or nausea;
- result of disruptions to your routine due to care;
- consequence of stress, depression or anxiety.

Many of these can affect the sleep of carers as well as the person with cancer. In some cases, your cancer team can help, perhaps by adjusting your treatment. Hypnotics (sleeping pills) and insomnia treatments you buy without a prescription can help re-establish a normal sleep pattern, but they are only a short-term fix until the good sleep hygiene tips in the box 'The principles of good sleep hygiene' work. (Both people with cancer and their carers should follow these tips.) Either way, do not suffer in silence.

The principles of good sleep hygiene

- Although regular exercise helps you sleep and counter cancer-related fatigue, exercising just before bed can disrupt sleep.
- If you experience cancer-related fatigue, you should schedule rest regularly throughout the day. Try to avoid naps, however, as they can make sleeping at night more difficult.
- Avoid alcohol. A nightcap can help you fall asleep, but as blood alcohol levels fall, sleep becomes more fragmented and lighter, so you might wake repeatedly in the latter part of the night.
- Avoid stimulants, such as caffeine and nicotine, for several hours before bed. Try hot milk or milky drinks instead.
- During the day you should remain hydrated, but do not drink too much fluid – even non-alcoholic – just before bed as this can mean regular trips to the bathroom.
- Do not eat a heavy meal before bedtime.
- Go to bed at the same time each night and set your alarm for the same time each morning, even at weekends. This helps re-establish a regular sleep pattern.
- Make the bed and bedroom as comfortable as possible. If you can afford to, invest in a comfortable mattress, with enough bedclothes. Make sure the room is not too hot, too cold or too bright. Try adding 'blackout' linings to curtains if too much light comes through them.
- Do not worry about anything you have forgotten to do. Simply jot it down – keep a notepad by the bed if you find you do this a lot – then get back to sleep. Making a note in this way should help you forget about the thing you need to remember until the morning.
- Although this is, for many people, a counsel of perfection, try not to take your troubles to bed with you. Brooding makes things seem worse, exacerbates stress, keeps you awake and, because you are tired in the morning, means you are less able to deal with your difficulties. If you can, avoid heavy conversations and arguments before bed.
- Use the bed for sex and sleep only. Do not work or watch television.

Self-help tips for sleep disturbance

Follow the sleep hygiene tips in the box 'The principles of good sleep hygiene', but if you still cannot sleep, get up and do something else. Watch the television or read – nothing too stimulating – until you feel tired. Lying there worrying about not sleeping keeps you awake.

Pain

Pain is often cancer's most feared symptom. Certainly, pain potentially undermines almost every aspect of your life – your day-to-day mood, your will to live, your relationships and social life, your ability to sleep, exercise and eat.[83] After all, pain is a biological alarm that evolved to warn you something's wrong, which is why it can be so hard to ignore. Chronic pain can seem like a loud alarm that you cannot turn off.

Pain can have numerous causes, including the tumour, its treatments and the aftermath of an operation. Some diagnostic procedures can be uncomfortable or even painful. In addition:

- nurses administer many cancer treatments by infusion, which can cause pain, swelling and skin reactions around where the tube enters your vein (see page 60);
- severe mucositis (see page 108) can be very uncomfortable;
- some cancer drugs can cause pain in the joints and muscles;
- radiotherapy can cause sore, even painful skin reactions.

Unfortunately, pain does not always subside after treatment ends. A study that included people with a variety of cancers found that a fifth still reported pain at least two years after diagnosis.[90] There is no need to suffer this in silence, however. Modern painkillers (analgesics) and other treatments can almost always adequately control cancer-related pain.

Do not grin and bear pain

Make sure that your cancer team knows when and where the pain develops, as well as its severity. You could keep a diary. The team will also need to know the type of pain. A dull pain might have different causes and treatment from pins and needles, for example, even if they are equally unpleasant. So, note if the pain is dull and aching or sharp and stabbing. Does it feel like an electric shock or pins and needles? It is especially important to tell your cancer team if:[87]

- you experience pain in a new part of the body;
- the pain is getting worse or the painkillers do not seem to work as well as they did;
- you experience numbness, weakness and/or tingling;
- you lose sensation in any part of your body;
- you experience changes in your ability to control your bladder or bowel;
- the pain interferes with your daily life.

Your doctor will probably begin by trying to control your pain using 'simple' painkillers, such as aspirin and paracetamol. If these prove inadequate, mild opioids (codeine) might be tried. Finally, you might be offered the strong opioids, such as morphine. You are extremely unlikely to become addicted if you follow the cancer team's advice – they can reassure you if you are worried about dependence. Follow the team's advice for painkillers, but, as a rule, take them regularly – such as every three to six hours – or as the pain begins to emerge. 'Grinning and bearing' the pain means that analgesics typically take longer to work.

Sometimes an operation or radiotherapy can alleviate pain. For example, surgeons or radiotherapy might remove or shrink a tumour that presses on a nerve. Surgeons can also cut certain nerves that carry the pain signal. Many people find that CAMs – such as hypnosis, acupuncture and massage – help control pain, but check with the cancer team first.

Self-help tips for alleviating peripheral neuropathy

Some drugs and certain malignancies might damage nerves, which can lead to peripheral neuropathy. Tell your cancer team if you develop symptoms such as:

- numbing, tingling or loss of feeling in the limbs;
- feeling as if you are wearing a sock or glove;
- burning, stabbing or electric shock-like pains;
- being very sensitive to touch.

Peripheral neuropathy seems to be most common with vinca alkaloids, taxanes and platinum derivatives. The longest nerves are the most susceptible, which is why peripheral neuropathy usually affects the hands and feet. Indeed, severe peripheral neuropathy can undermine movement. Cisplatin can also damage nerves involved in hearing, which might cause partial deafness and tinnitus (ringing in the ears). In general, peripheral neuropathy abates over several months once treatment ends. Occasionally, however, symptoms persist for months or even years after your last course of chemotherapy.[2, 3]

In the meantime, analgesics and some other drugs might help. Some people find that avoiding alcohol and, as far as possible, repetitive activities that might stress nerves – such as golf, tennis, playing an instrument or using a computer keyboard – alleviates the discomfort. Some also benefit from CAMs, such as biofeedback, acupuncture, hypnosis and relaxation techniques.[87]

Self-help tips for muscle and joint pain

Some chemotherapies – including taxanes and vinca alkaloids – and certain cancers can cause painful joints (arthralgia) and muscles (myalgia). Often simple painkillers help. In addition, you could:[87]

- apply a heat pad, hot water bottle, an ice pack or a packet of frozen peas to the painful joint or muscle;
- soak in a warm bath (check with your cancer team before using aromatherapy essences as some might not be suitable and you need to make sure anything you add to your bath will not undermine your skin care);
- try massage, acupuncture, hypnosis and relaxation techniques.

Skin, hair and nails

Skin, hair and nail cells divide rapidly. You replace about 30,000 skin cells every minute, for instance.[7] So, as with any rapidly dividing tissue, cancer treatment can take its toll on your skin, nails and hair.

Some cancer drugs, for example, might cause an area of dry, scaly skin. Some might trigger an itchy, red area. Others might cause pus-filled pimples that look like acne. Radiotherapy can mean that your skin blisters and peels, leaving moist red areas.[91] Your cancer team can suggest steroids, antibiotics and other drugs that might help protect and heal your skin, and dressings that should speed the healing of any damage following radiotherapy.[91] Mention any change in your skin to your cancer team.

Self-help tips for looking after your skin

You can take several steps to care for your skin.[91]

- If you develop a skin reaction or have received radiotherapy, check which creams, cosmetics, medicines, tapes and plasters, and bath products you can use and ask if you should change any.
- Do not use perfumed soap, skincare products, cosmetics or deodorants.
- Use a moisturizer regularly on dry skin. Check with the cancer team or radiotherapist which is the best one for you to use. You can swim after checking with the cancer team, but chlorine can dry skin, so use a moisturizer.
- Avoid long hot showers and baths. Wash in warm or tepid water and do not stay in too long.
- Pat yourself dry with a clean, smooth towel. Do not rub.
- Make sure the house is not too warm and try a humidifier if the air seems dry.
- Avoid wool and synthetic fibres. Wear loose-fitting, soft cotton clothes. Wash sheets and clothing in mild detergents.
- Avoid wet shaving. Do not use hair-removal creams or wax, especially on the area being treated.
- If you develop diarrhoea, be particularly careful about personal hygiene: chemicals in faeces can damage the delicate skin around the anus.

Self-help tips for protecting your skin

Your skin and the sun

Safe sun practices prevent most skin cancers, but you need to remain vigilant, especially if you are taking certain cancer treatments or have already had a skin malignancy. For example:[94]

- three-fifths (60 per cent) of people who have their first non-melanoma skin cancer develop another of these malignancies within ten years;
- if it is not their first, a similar proportion (62 per cent) develop another non-melanoma skin cancer within two years;

- if it is not their first, 9 in 10 (91 per cent) develop another non-melanoma skin cancer within a decade.

So keep an eye out for any changes to your skin. Examine your skin every month: a check only takes ten minutes or so. Take a selfie, use mirrors or ask a friend or family member to look at 'difficult to view' skin areas. You could mark the location of each mole, birthmark, bump, sore, scaly patch and so on on an outline of the body (<www.skincancer.org/skin-cancer-information/early-detection/body-map>) to help you identify any changes.

Your cancer team can tell you what to watch for, but if you are unsure, check and tell them or your GP if you see any of the following:

- a lesion (such as a spot, blemish or mole) that is growing, bleeding, changing in appearance or never heals completely;
- a discoloured red, scaly patch on the skin that might itch;
- an irregularly shaped new mole or an existing mole that changes shape.

Radiotherapy and some cancer treatments can leave your skin highly sensitive to the sun – so-called photosensitivity reactions. This means that you are much more likely to burn than you were before treatment. With some treatments the skin might be so sensitive that you get sunburn even indoors – through windows – or on cloudy days.[91] So you might have to use suncream on cloudy days and during the winter. Ask your cancer team about the precautions you need to take.

You should also ask your cancer team for advice about the right sun protection factor (SPF) and sunscreen for you, but as a general rule, apply suncream with a SPF of 15 or more at least every two hours. Apply the suncream more frequently if you are sweating or swimming. Some people will need a minimum SPF of 30 and ideally 50, either because of a malignancy (in those who have had a skin cancer, for example) or its treatment (drugs that cause photosensitivity reactions, for instance).

Cover as much skin as possible, including your ears and any bald patches, and use a lip balm. In addition:

- wear a broad-brimmed hat, UV-protective sunglasses and clothing with a close weave that covers as much skin as possible;

- wear UV-protective swim- and beachwear;
- avoid direct sunlight as much as possible, especially from 11 a.m. to 3 p.m.;
- if you are particularly photosensitive, consider using window films that block UV in the home, office and car;
- avoid sunbeds or sunlamps.

Your skin and radiotherapy

If you are receiving radiotherapy, skin reactions usually begin about a week after the start of the treatment, peak about a week after the radiotherapy ends and generally take two to six weeks to resolve. Fortunately, long-term effects on the skin are uncommon.[3] To reduce skin damage during radiotherapy, try the tips listed below:[3]

- avoid friction, from towels or tight-fitting clothes, for example;
- avoid chemical irritants, such as perfumes, powders and deodorants;
- avoid using razor blades;
- avoid excessive heat and cold during treatment by, for example, showering in warm water;
- wash with mild soap;
- do not use oils or lotions;
- dry skin might respond to emollients, moisturizers or aloe vera gel;
- tell your cancer team if you see a wound on your skin – several specialized wound dressings can aid healing;
- tell your cancer team if you feel that your skin is itching.

Your skin and itchiness

Once again, cancer-related itchiness has several causes. For example, a cancer can release chemicals that trigger this. Often the irritation subsides if treatment shrinks the cancer. In other cases your bile duct can become blocked by a tumour. The build-up of bilirubin and other toxins can cause itchiness. Surgeons might be able to unblock a blocked bile duct or a doctor can prescribe a drug called cholestyramine, which binds the itch-promoting bile salts.

Your cancer team might suggest antihistamines. These block the action of histamine, a chemical messenger that triggers itchiness. Low doses of some drugs (used – at higher doses – to treat depression or epilepsy) might be especially helpful if peripheral neuropathy or other forms of nerve irritation are causing the itch. Doctors can also prescribe steroids as creams or tablets. These dampen the activity of the cells that trigger itchiness.

Contact your cancer team if:

- the itching worsens or becomes more widespread;
- an itchy area of skin becomes redder and sore, leaks pus or smells;
- you cannot sleep because of the itch;
- the treatments do not seem to be working.

Listed below are some self-help tips that might help you deal with itchy skin.

- Several CAMs – including acupuncture, hypnosis or relaxation therapy – may alleviate the intensity of the itch.
- Apply a cold pack or a packet of frozen peas to the itchy area. Some people find that rubbing, tapping or pressing the itchy area or gently pinching nearby skin helps.
- Apply an unscented and colourless moisturizer after bathing or when the itching is uncomfortable. Ask your cancer team or a pharmacist which is the best one for you to use.
- Do not take too many baths, do not spend longer than about 20 minutes in the bath and use lukewarm water.
- Use little or no soap; try a bathtime emollient suggested by your doctor, pharmacist or nurse instead.
- Some people find oatmeal baths help.
- Pat skin dry with a towel rather than rub it – but dry yourself well to help reduce chafing and the risk of fungal infections.
- Drink 2–3 litres of fluid a day – dehydration can trigger or exacerbate itchiness.
- Keep rooms cool and humid – hot and dry atmospheres can make itchiness worse.
- Keeping your nails short and wearing soft cotton mittens and socks may help prevent skin damage if you cannot stop scratching, especially in your sleep.
- Avoid things that might make your itch worse, such as certain hair and cleaning products, scented products or preparations containing lanolin.
- Wearing loose-fitting cotton clothes often helps – wool and man-made fabrics can irritate the skin.

- Try to take your mind off the itch by watching television, listening to music, reading or whatever else distracts you.

Self-help tips for nails

People spend millions each year on manicures, false nails and polishes to make their nails attractive. Nails also protect your fingertips and, by supporting the other side of the finger, help you make precise, delicate movements and enhance the sensitivity of your touch.

Many people receiving chemotherapy find that their nails grow more slowly than usual and become fragile and brittle. The nails might lift from the bed and break easily or develop horizontal lines (Beau's lines).[3] Watch for any changes, such as separation of the nail from the nail bed, discolouration or an increase in milk spots.

The following tips might help to keep your nails in as good a condition as possible:

- use a moisturizer regularly;
- wear gloves, which helps protect delicate nails;
- do not use false nails;
- keep your nails short, but do not push back the cuticle, which can increase the risk of infections, and do not have aggressive manicures or pedicures or bite your nails;
- keep your hands and feet as dry as possible.

In general, nail symptoms resolve when treatment ends, but see your cancer team if you are experiencing pain or performing normal activities becomes more difficult.

Self-help tips for protecting your hair

Hair loss (alopecia) is, perhaps, the most familiar side effect of cancer treatment and can cause considerable distress.[3]

Healthy head hair grows by approximately 12 cm (5 inches) a year and you normally lose about 100 hairs a day. As we have seen, chemo- and radiotherapy target rapidly dividing cells, so losing a few more hairs is common during treatment for cancer. Do not worry, though, if you see a few extra hairs on our brush – you need to lose at least half your hair before anyone else will notice.[87]

Hair loss typically starts to happen two to three weeks after the first chemo- or radiotherapy treatment has been given, usually beginning on the crown and above the ears. In addition to scalp hair, you can lose beard, eyebrows and pubic and body hair.

Radiotherapy, especially to the brain and head, can cause hair loss. Hair regrowth following radiotherapy can be extremely slow and might be incomplete. Unless you have received very high levels of radiotherapy, hair normally grows back within three to five months of the end of treatment.

Sometimes regrowth begins before chemotherapy ends, but it might curl as it pushes through the scalp – sometimes called 'chemo curl' – and might be a different texture or colour than it was before treatment.[3, 87]

Speak to your cancer team, a counsellor or a patient support group if your hair loss causes you distress. The tips given below might help limit the impact:

- cut your hair short when you start treatment – any loss might seem less dramatic and you will regain your style more quickly afterwards;
- hair loss can leave skin sensitive or tender, even before the loss becomes visible, so be careful if you shave, depilate or cut hair anywhere on your body;
- massaging the scalp removes dry skin and flakes;
- do not wash your hair every day and use mild or baby shampoo when you do;
- do not scrub your hair dry vigorously – gently pat your hair dry;
- brush your hair gently using a soft hairbrush, especially when it begins to regrow, and limit pinning, curling or blow-drying your hair at a high heat setting;
- avoid using chemicals (such as hair colour) until your hair has regrown and, if you do, test any chemical on a small patch of hair first and avoid hair colour for at least three months after your treatment ends;
- choose a soft, comfortable covering for the bed pillow;
- think about a wig or hairpiece – a hairdresser can help you style the wig or hairpiece, which you should have fitted properly to stop scalp irritation;
- you could try wearing some form of comfortable hat or other head covering.

Cold capping might help. A coolant at around –5 °C (23 °F) is circulated around a special head piece before, during and after chemotherapy. The cold reduces blood flow to the scalp, which means that less of the drug reaches the rapidly dividing cells that produce the hair. Cold capping does not always work and some people find the experience unpleasant, but it does help some people keep their hair.[3] Ask your cancer team if you want to know more.

Anorexia and cachexia

Up to 2 in 5 (40 per cent) of people with cancer overall and as many as 7 in 10 (70 per cent) of those with advanced cancer experience poor appetite and unintentional weight loss (anorexia).[87] Cachexia (wasting of fat and muscle), which eventually emerges in up to half of people with cancer, usually develops slowly, beginning with weight loss over several months.[95] Anorexia, weight loss and cachexia undermine people's ability to cope with everyday activities, worsen quality of life, can reduce the effectiveness of some treatments and may shorten survival.[87, 95]

Several factors contribute to anorexia, weight loss and cachexia in people with cancer, including those listed below.

- The site of the tumour can play a role. For example, people with oesophageal, stomach, pancreatic and small cell lung cancers seem to be at especially high risk. Tumours in the oesophagus, for example, can leave the person feeling as if food is stuck in the throat and 4 in 5 patients with stomach or pancreatic cancer, 3 in 5 with lung or prostate cancer and 1 in 3 of those with breast cancer show marked weight loss over six months.[83, 87, 95]
- Between 5 and 9 in 10 people with advanced cancer report changes in taste and smell (see below), which, if severe, can put people off their food.[83]
- Depression, anxiety, constipation, dry mouth, mucositis (pain and inflammation of the lining of the gastrointestinal tract – see below), nausea and vomiting can make eating difficult.[83]
- Some medicines (for cancer and some other diseases) or radiotherapy result in a dry mouth (see below).[36]

It is important to speak to your cancer team. Managing symptoms and side effects, and making changes to your diet – including using nutritional supplements if appropriate – usually helps. In addition, light exercise an hour or two before eating can sharpen the appetite.[83] You could walk around the block, for example.

People with cancer often feel full sooner than when they were healthy and may find eating five or six small meals a day easier than having three larger meals. Try to eat one or two of these meals with your family. If you cannot finish and your family is worried, remind them that you are eating more frequently. Keep healthy snacks – such as carrot sticks, slices of sweet peppers, fresh and dried fruits – by you for when you feel peckish.[83]

Self-help tips for dealing with changes in senses of taste and smell

Many people with cancer find their senses of taste and smell change. This can arise, for example, as a symptom of head and neck cancer[96] or as a side effect of radiotherapy to some parts of the body. Taste usually returns two to three months after radiotherapy ends.[3]

Taste changes seem to be especially common with chemotherapy: more than half (38–84 per cent in different studies) of patients receiving chemotherapy develop taste changes.[96, 97] How many experience changes in their sense of smell due to chemotherapy is less clear.[96] Many people with cancer – perhaps 1 in 10 (10 per cent) to three quarters (78 per cent) – report a metallic taste in their mouths.[96, 97]

The likelihood of developing taste changes depends on the drug used and may arise, for example, due to:

- changes in saliva and mucus production – some antidepressants, antihistamines and diuretics (water tablets) reduce saliva production leading to a dry mouth;
- certain drugs reaching the mouth from the blood;
- damage to the cells and nerves that detect taste.

Often the sense of taste returns once chemotherapy ends,[96] but you should tell the cancer team if you experience changes. In one study, about a third of patients reported a metallic taste. The oncologist was aware of the change in only about 1 in 10 cases.[97]

If you experience changes in your senses of taste and smell, the tips listed below may help (you might need to try more than one):[3, 96, 97]

- using plastic rather than metallic cutlery;
- consuming cold or frozen drinks and food (such as iced water and lollies) often helps people with metallic taste alterations, but not those who experience changes with their perception of salty tastes;
- eating food at room temperature;
- adding strong herbs or spices to food, but some people find reducing seasoning helps, so experiment to discover what is right for you;
- marinating meat with fruit juice, wine, cider or adding sweeteners or acid (such as citrus fruits and vinegar) to food;
- try *Synsepalum dulcificum* – sometimes called the 'miracle fruit' or 'miracle berry' – but always check with the cancer team before taking any herbal supplement (chemicals in the miracle fruit seem to make sour food taste sweet and, in small studies, some people receiving chemotherapy found that *S. dulcificum* helps with the metallic taste);
- eating sweet-and-sour foods;
- a metallic or bitter taste on eating red meat is probably caused by the iron in it, so choose from other sources of protein, such as fish, poultry, eggs, cheese, soya and dairy (you may need to take a supplement to maintain your iron stores – check with your cancer team).

Self-help tips for dealing with mucositis and stomatitis

Between 2 and 5 in every 10 people who receive chemotherapy develop mucositis – pain and inflammation of the layer of tissue that lines the gastrointestinal tract from the mouth to the anus. Stomatitis refers to mucositis in the mouth. Up to half of people receiving both chemotherapy and radiotherapy develop mucositis. Indeed, mucositis and stomatitis are almost inevitable with chemotherapy and radiotherapy for cancers of the head and neck, and are very common after bone marrow transplants.[2, 87, 91]

Mucositis usually develops 7–14 days after treatment begins and typically lasts for 2–3 weeks after treatment ends. Mucositis and stomatitis might leave you susceptible to oral thrush (oral candidiasis), a fungal infection that causes uncomfortable white patches on the mouth and tongue. Candidiasis can lead to a loss of taste or there being an unpleasant taste in the mouth.[87, 91]

Speak to your cancer team if you develop any of these symptoms, which could arise from mucositis:

- dry, cracked lips;
- pain;
- difficulties swallowing;
- ulcers and sores on the mouth and tongue;
- bleeding.

Bleeding gums

Some malignancies and cancer treatments can affect platelets (the blood cells responsible for clots), so contact your cancer team if you bleed excessively when you brush or floss. A dental check-up before starting cancer treatment can help address any issues that could get worse during treatment.[91]

Severe mucositis might need potent painkillers, intravenous fluids and tube feeding. Mouthwashes, less potent painkillers and barrier products can help with milder symptoms.[3, 85–87, 91] In addition, you could take the following steps to relieve symptoms.[3]

- Rinse your mouth out with warm water with a little salt dissolved in it, sterile water or a non-alcoholic, unsweetened mouthwash after each meal and at bedtime. You could rinse with 1 teaspoon of salt or 1–2 teaspoons of baking soda in a litre of water. If you want to rinse more often, check which mouthwash to use and how often you should use it with your cancer team or dentist, who might be able to suggest mouthwashes that reduce the pain and inflammation.
- Gently brush and floss at least twice a day unless your doctor tells you otherwise. Use teeth sponges and a soft – or a child's – toothbrush to clean your teeth; this helps reduce gum damage. You might find that a toothpaste for sensitive teeth is more comfortable than your usual brand.
- Zinc supplements (220 mg zinc sulphate twice daily) can reduce the severity of mucositis. Again, always check with your cancer team before taking supplements.
- The mouth is susceptible to fungal infections, such as thrush. Rinsing reduces the risk, but tell your cancer team if you notice any white patches. Antifungals can treat thrush infections.

- Tell your cancer team if your mouth is painful. A change to your painkillers often helps.
- Some people find that sucking ice cubes or an ice lolly alleviates the discomfort. You could also try this during chemotherapy – the approach is similar to using a cold cap to reduce alopecia.[2]
- A vitamin E supplement and 'swish and swallow' formulations of glutamine might reduce the frequency, severity and duration of oral mucositis. Tablets and other oral formulations of glutamine do not seem to be as effective as swish and swallow.
- Ask your cancer team about these and other antiseptic and anti-inflammatory mouthwashes, gels and so on. Your pharmacist or cancer team can suggest treatments for mouth ulcers and sores.
- Vaseline or a lip balm might ease sore lips.
- Avoid spicy, salty or acidic foods, as well as raw vegetables, granola, toast and other 'rough' foods. If hot and warm foods irritate your mouth, eat cold foods or meals at room temperature. Try eating soft food, such as mashed potatoes, scrambled eggs, macaroni cheese, cottage cheese, soft fruits or purées, soups, milk and yogurt shakes.
- If you want to drink alcohol, avoid neat spirits. Some people find that tomato, grapefruit and some orange juices irritate their mouths. Drink plenty of water, if necessary using a straw or a bottle with a sports cap.

Self-help tips for a dry mouth

Apart from being uncomfortable, a dry mouth (xerostomia) can make speaking, chewing and swallowing difficult and can lead to, for example, halitosis (bad breath), recurrent mouth infections (including thrush), taste changes, tooth decay and gum disease.[3, 91]

Once again, dry mouth can arise from several causes – radiotherapy, for instance, can damage your salivary glands. In general, salivary glands start working properly three to four months after the end of radiotherapy, but if you received a large dose of radiation, dry mouth might last longer or even be permanent.[91] Several cancers, certain drugs and dehydration can reduce saliva production.

If you develop dry mouth, try the tips given below, which might help (you may need to try more than one):[3, 91]

- avoid dry foods, such as biscuits, crackers and breads;
- choose recipes and food with plenty of gravy, sauces, cream and butter;
- sip on liquids throughout the day;
- rinse your mouth out with a teaspoon of baking soda (sodium bicarbonate) dissolved in a glass of warm water;
- chew or suck gums, sweets, pastilles or pineapple chunks;
- avoid dry foods such as crackers, flaky pastry and chocolate – these can stick to the lining of the mouth;
- regularly sip cold water or unsweetened drinks – some people find that fizzy drinks are better for a dry mouth than still drinks;
- smear your mouth and tongue with olive oil or melted butter – some people find that this helps especially at night;
- cut out smoking and alcohol (including mouth washes containing alcohol) and, for some people, tea and coffee – all these can dry the mouth;
- suck ice cubes and lollies.

If these do not help enough, speak to your cancer team, who can prescribe artificial saliva – which comes as a spray, gel or lozenge – and other products to help a dry mouth. Sometimes a change in drugs can help. You can use artificial saliva before and during meals.

Your cancer team or GP can prescribe a drug called pilocarpine, which might stimulate glands that have been damaged by radiotherapy to produce more saliva. Some people also find that acupuncture relieves their symptoms.[3, 91]

Lymphoedema

Sometimes damage to, or removal of parts of the lymphatic system (see page 7) can lead to fluid retention and tissue swelling. This reaction, called lymphoedema, causes swelling, usually in the limbs. The swelling may, however, extend to the groin, face, neck and genitals.

Lymphoedema can impair body image, sexuality, social activities and your ability to perform some jobs or activities around the house.[87]

Self-help tips for lymphoedema

If you develop lymphoedema, try one or more of the following strategies, which might help:[87]

- many people find that strengthening and aerobic exercises are especially helpful, but avoid heavy lifting (more than about 7 kilos/15 lbs) or vigorous repetitive movements against resistance;
- be careful not to injure parts of the body affected by lymphoedema;
- ensure good hygiene to prevent infections;
- watch for any signs of an infection – such as a raised temperature – and speak to your GP or cancer team if you think you might have one;
- avoid keeping a swollen leg still for a long time, such as during a flight or car journey;
- try to maintain a healthy weight;
- eat a low-salt, high-fibre diet, which helps remove excess fluids.

Pyrexia

Some cancers and certain treatments can increase the chance of catching a viral, fungal or bacterial infection. Pyrexia (a high temperature) is part of the body's natural response to infections. In addition, some cancers release chemicals that cause fever.

Pyrexia usually passes as your body adjusts – a bit like resetting the thermostat on your central heating. In the meantime, drugs such as paracetamol, ibuprofen or aspirin can help bring your temperature down and alleviate any pain and discomfort. You might need to take doses every four to six hours until your temperature returns to normal. Ask your cancer team which drug is best for you. You should not take aspirin, however, if, for example, you have a low count of platelets or are at risk of bleeding for other reasons.

Contact your GP or cancer team urgently if you:

- feel very unwell or your temperature is very high – such as over 39.4 °C (103 °F);
- your temperature does not return to normal after a couple of days;
- you feel faint and lightheaded, which might be a sign that your blood pressure is low;
- you feel confused or very agitated;
- you feel very drowsy.

Self-help tips for pyrexia

Try the tips listed below individually or in combination to lower your temperature:

- remove excess clothing and bedlinen;
- have tepid baths, showers or sponge yourself down with tepid or cool water;
- drink lots of cold fluids;
- suck on ice cubes or ice lollies;
- open the window or have a fan in the room;
- rest;
- if you experience chills (feeling cold when there isn't an obvious cause), change any wet bedlinen and clothes, stay away from draughts and keep windows closed, but, if your temperature is still high, avoid the temptation to huddle up under a blanket – you could make the fever worse or it may last longer.

Menopausal symptoms

Some drugs and hormonal treatments can cause 'menopausal' symptoms, including:[87]

- changes to the pattern of, or the end of periods – fourth-fifths of women who are less than 25 years of age recover their normal menstrual cycles after chemotherapy ends; women who are more than 40 years of age are at higher risk of permanent menopause;
- forgetfulness and poor concentration;
- hot flushes;
- mood changes;
- night sweats;
- sleep disturbances;
- urinary incontinence;
- vaginal dryness.

Men taking hormonal treatments, such as for prostate cancer, can experience some 'menopausal' symptoms, including hot flushes, sweating and breast tenderness. Doctors can prescribe drugs that can alleviate some of these symptoms.

Self-help tips for menopausal symptoms

You could try the suggestions given below, which may help to alleviate menopausal symptoms:

- a low-fat diet, which might reduce the severity and frequency of menopausal symptoms;[87]
- avoiding spicy foods, caffeine and excessive amounts of alcohol, which might reduce hot flushes;
- vitamin E might reduce the number of hot flushes triggered by hormonal treatments;[12]
- relaxation, acupuncture, quitting smoking, maintaining a healthy weight and regular exercise might reduce the severity and frequency of menopausal symptoms.[87]

Self-help tips for hot flushes

Between 3 and 4 in 10 (30 and 40 per cent) of women with breast cancer experience persistent moderate to severe hot flushes. The sensation of intense heat begins, usually, in the chest then moves to the neck and face. Women might flush, sweat and experience heart palpitations. The symptoms typically last from several seconds to a few minutes. Hot flushes at night often disrupt sleep.[98]

Tell your cancer team if you experience hot flushes. Some drugs – including certain medicines used to treat depression – alleviate severe hot flushes, whether or not you experience mood disturbances. Indeed, antidepressants seem to reduce the frequency and severity of hot flushes in women with breast cancer by up to two-fifths (14–58 per cent) compared to an inactive placebo. Antidepressants used to treat hot flushes might cause side effects, however – including dry mouth, headache, constipation, nausea and loss of appetite – and might interact with other drugs you are taking for cancer and other ailments.[99]

There are several other approaches that might help:[98, 99]

- dressing in layers so you can keep cool;
- cool drinks and food;
- using a fan;
- drinking less caffeine and eating fewer meals with hot spices;
- avoiding hot rooms and hot baths;
- stopping smoking;

- keeping a healthy weight;
- taking regular exercise;
- reducing stress – try relaxation techniques and other CAMs after checking with your cancer team;
- several studies, mainly of women with breast cancer, report that acupuncture reduces the severity and frequency of hot flushes, and, in many cases, sleep seemed to improve as the hot flushes abated.

Some people feel that eating foods rich in phyto-oestrogens and related chemicals called isoflavones – such as soy, chickpeas, mung beans, flax seeds and alfalfa sprouts – alleviates hot flushes. (Phyto-oestrogens are chemicals produced by plants that resemble the hormone and so bind to the same receptors – see page 66.) You can also buy phyto-oestrogen supplements. Several studies have assessed various formulations of phyto-oestrogens for hot flushes (among women undergoing treatment for breast cancer, for example), but there is currently little evidence that phyto-oestrogens reduce the risk compared to placebo.[99] That said, foods rich in phyto-oestrogens are generally healthy, so you could always try them, after checking with your cancer team first. After all, phyto-oestrogens act as mild hormones, which means high doses of phyto-oestrogens might not be suitable for people with some hormone-sensitive cancers.

Sexual difficulties

Sexual issues and worries about sexual performance associated with cancer and its treatment can cause considerable stress and affect relationships. Sexual difficulties might arise from:

- changes in body image;
- anxiety and depression;
- physical symptoms, such as vaginal dryness and erectile dysfunction (impotence).[3]

At least half of people with breast, prostate, colorectal and gynaecological cancers endure long-term sexual difficulties.[87] For instance, 2 in 5 (42 per cent) of prostate cancer survivors and 1 in 5 (20 per cent) of breast cancer survivors reported changes in sexual interest. About half (46 per cent) of prostate cancer survivors and a third (31 per cent) of men with colorectal cancer experience erectile dysfunction.[3] Despite being common, many people suffer in silence. Don't. Speak to your cancer team – there's often a lot they can do to help.

Effects on fertility

You should consider any impact on sexuality or fertility when deciding on treatment. Chemotherapy – especially combination treatment – can impair fertility, for example. The effects depend on the drug. Vinca alkaloids and anthracyclines tend to produce a short-lived reduction in sperm production, for example, while other drugs – such as cyclophosphamide and cisplatin – can reduce sperm counts for much longer.[3] Regimens containing alkylating agents – such as those used to treat Hodgkin's lymphoma – can cause sterility in 4 in 5 men (80 per cent) and 1 in 2 (50 per cent) women.[2] Sperm take about 72 days to develop,[100] so sperm counts typically decline over 2–3 months.[2] In women, chemotherapy tends to reduce the number of viable oocytes (the cells that develop into eggs).[3]

If you want to start a family or have more children, ask about sperm banking or egg storage.[87] Also, check when it is safe to have penetrative sex, especially if you have brachytherapy, surgery or radiotherapy to your pelvis.[91]

Radiotherapy to the pelvis can cause adhesions (bands of scars) that narrow or shorten the vagina. If you are having radiotherapy to the vagina, you can use a vaginal dilator, which is shaped like a tampon, to stretch the vagina, prevent adhesions and break up scar tissue. Regular sex also helps.[91]

Self-help tips to give your sex life a boost

Try the tips listed below, which may help.[87]

- Fatigue can mean you feel too worn out to have sex – try the tips given on page 92.
- Avoid large meals if you think you are likely to have sex. Digestion diverts blood from other parts of your body – including your sexual organs – to your gut.
- Change position – your partner being on top can help prevent breathlessness or might relieve the pressure on sore parts of your body.

- Non-irritating lubricants – ask your pharmacist or cancer team – can help if you experience vaginal dryness.
- Living with stress, anxiety, depression and altered body image can affect desire and libido. If you get an erection during the night or in the morning, the cause might be more psychological than physiological. Relaxation, anti-stress techniques and advice from a counsellor or a patient group can often help if stress undermines your sex drive.
- Doctors can prescribe several drugs to help with impotence, but never buy any drug online. If you want to try a herbal treatment for impotence, check with your cancer team first to ensure that it does not interact with your treatment.
- Several drugs that lower blood pressure, certain treatments for depression and anxiety, and some other medicines can cause impotence. If you think that a drug might be causing or contributing to your dificulties, speak to your doctor – there is usually an alternative.
- Avoid anything that triggers nausea, which might include perfumes, aftershaves, scented candles and so on. Having a light snack before you expect to have sex could help by settling your stomach.
- Pain can make sex difficult. Take painkillers an hour before if you expect to have sex, try different positions and support painful areas with cushions or pillows.

How partners can help

Partners of people with cancer can also help give their sex life a boost.

- Spend time with your partner or go on 'dates'. Some carers find that the increased opportunity to be intimate when looking after a survivor increases sexual desire. Consider making time with your partner a 'priority' when planning to cope with fatigue.
- Reassure your partner that you love and find him or her attractive despite any physical changes or side effects or having to care for physical needs.
- Discuss any fears or concerns you have about being intimate with your partner. If necessary, swallow your embarrassment and speak to the cancer team, a patient support group or a counsellor.

They can reassure you if, for example, you are worried that being intimate might cause the cancer survivor pain.

- Be patient. It might take a few weeks for a person with cancer to get his or her sexual confidence back.
- Keep an open mind. You might have to find new ways to make love, such as being more forward, becoming the 'dominant' partner or using sex toys and lubricants. Sexual pleasure is not always about penetration; it is also about intimacy.

Talk to your cancer team, a counsellor or a patient support group if you feel these approaches are not making a difference.

Depression and anxiety

Is it any wonder that people with cancer feel depressed about the cancer attacking their bodies? Is it any wonder they feel anxious about being a burden to their families or friends, the cancer recurring or financial difficulties? That so many people with cancer *do not* develop profound depression or anxiety amazes me. Some even manage to use their adversity as a springboard to personal growth.

Nevertheless, depression is common among people with cancer. In addition, brain tumours or metastases can cause psychiatric symptoms, such as depression, mania, hallucinations, anxiety or anorexia nervosa. Indeed, depression might be the only sign of a brain tumour.[101] That is another reason why people with cancer need to get new or worsening depression checked.

More than a low mood

Depression is much more debilitating, intrusive and distressing than a low mood or the 'simple' sadness that is natural when you face a life-transforming event, such as cancer. Depression is a profound, debilitating mental and physical lethargy, which is why it can make fatigue worse; a pervasive sense of worthlessness, despite evidence to the contrary; an intense, deep, unshakable, guilt and crushing sadness. As William Styron remarks in *Darkness Visible*, depression 'remains nearly incomprehensible to those who have not experienced it in its extreme mode'.

The symptoms of depression differ from person to person. Nevertheless, doctors recognize several core symptoms. People with depression typically spend a considerable time ruminating about the past, for example, and feel guilty about mistakes, when they let others down and events and acts they regard as immoral or sinful. Some patients and carers might develop depression because they regard the cancer as 'punishment' for their sins.

When to see your doctor

The more of the symptoms listed in the box 'Examples of the core symptoms of depression' you have, the more likely you are to have depression, especially if they persist and interfere with your day-to-day life. See your GP as soon as you can if you have little interest or take little pleasure in doing things you used to enjoy or you feel down, depressed or hopeless for most of the day, every day, for more than two weeks. See your doctor *urgently* if:

- you feel that life is unbearable;
- you are considering or taking steps towards suicide or self-harming;
- you cannot meet your work, social and family obligations;
- you lack the motivation to work towards your goals, to exercise or follow your treatment or fatigue plan;
- you hear voices in your head – which are usually critical or defamatory – or experience visual hallucinations (hallucinations can be symptoms of a very serious condition called psychotic depression; in addition, some brain cancers and certain medicines can trigger hallucinations).

Tragically, cancer patients are more likely to die as a result of suicide than those without a malignancy. Researchers combined results from 15 studies looking at the risk and presented their findings at the European Congress of Psychiatry in 2017. Cancer patients were half as much again (55 per cent) more likely to commit suicide than the general population or to die from suicide than from other causes (53 per cent), such as a traffic accident or sudden heart attack.

If you feel suicidal or are getting to the end of your tether, then see your GP, go to the accident and emergency department of your local hospital, speak to your cancer team or phone a helpline, such as:

- Samaritans 116 123
- Breathing Space 0800 83 85 87
- HOPElineUK: 0800 068 41 41.

Examples of the core symptoms of depression

Examples of the psychological symptoms of depression

- Considering suicide, self-harm or taking steps towards suicide.
- Continuous low mood or sadness.
- Feeling anxious or worried.
- Feeling hopeless and helpless.
- Feeling irritable and intolerant of others.
- Feeling guilty – especially if the guilt is excessive or unjustified.
- Feeling tearful or crying.
- Lack of interest in things or activities – especially if these were once important or enjoyable.
- Lacking motivation.
- Low self-esteem.
- Procrastination – finding it difficult to make decisions.

Examples of the physical symptoms of depression

- Change in appetite or weight (usually loss of weight, but can be weight gain).
- Changes to the menstrual cycle.
- Constipation.
- Feeling lethargic – moving more slowly than usual.
- Lack of energy.
- Loss of libido.
- Sleep disturbances, such as difficulty falling asleep at night or waking early in the morning.
- Speaking more slowly or less than usual.
- Unexplained aches and pains.

Examples of the social symptoms of depression

- Avoiding contact with friends and family.
- Avoiding social activities.
- Neglecting and not being interested in your hobbies and interests.
- Poor performance at work, such as poor concentration, lack of motivation, absenteeism.
- Issues in your home and family life.

Adapted from NHS Choices.

Physical symptoms of depression

Depression affects the body, mind and emotions. For example, about two-thirds of people with depression develop somatic (physical) symptoms, such as:[102–104]

- aches and pains
- back pain, especially in the lower back
- breathing difficulty or breathlessness
- chest pains
- digestive symptoms – nausea, diarrhoea or constipation – and stomach pain
- dizziness, light-headedness or feeling faint
- headaches
- difficulty swallowing
- tiredness, exhaustion and fatigue.

These overlap with many symptoms of cancer or the side effects of certain treatments. Keeping a diary might help to distinguish symptoms of depression from those linked to the malignancy. For example, the aches and pains that arise as a somatic symptom of depression often seem to be 'everywhere' rather than affecting a specific part of the body, such as muscles or joints. You should always get any symptoms that are unpleasant, painful or limit your ability to perform the activities of daily living checked out.

Anxiety

Anxiety evolved to produce physical, mental and behavioural changes that warn us of, and help us deal with, potential dangers, such as walking alone late at night. Anxiety disorders arise when our natural 'fear' reaction is out of proportion to the threat, excessively prolonged or interferes with our everyday life.

Essentially, people with anxiety are highly sensitive to potential threats. Their enhanced fear response leaves them 'hyper-aroused' and sensitive. They might feel restless, panicky, on edge and irritable, and their heart may be racing or palpitating. They might have difficulty concentrating and sleeping, feel sweaty, dizzy, need to urinate a lot and suffer chest and abdominal pain.[87] People with anxiety usually recognize that their concern is excessive.

Answering 'yes' to either of the questions below suggests that you might have anxiety.[105]

- During the past four weeks, have you been bothered by feeling worried, tense or anxious most of the time?
- Are you frequently tense, irritable and having trouble sleeping?

Anxiety's physical symptoms

Anxiety increases mental alertness and heightens your senses to help you detect danger. Adrenaline and other chemicals flood your body. Your heartbeat increases; you breathe more rapidly; you sweat. Blood flows from your skin and your intestines to your muscles – that is why we go pale when stressed or frightened. Muscles surrounding the hair follicles tighten, causing goosebumps. The pupils dilate, so you are wide-eyed with fear.

This flood of chemicals can cause physical symptoms – hence phrases such as 'sick with fear', 'the runs' and 'butterflies in the tummy'. Anxiety also causes symptoms that overlap with those caused by some cancers and certain side effects, such as tense, sore

Post-traumatic stress disorder

People with cancer can develop post-traumatic stress disorder (PTSD) – the condition closely related to anxiety that also causes the shell shock endured by some of those in the armed services. Between 1 in 14 and 1 in 3 (7–35 per cent) people with breast cancer seem to develop symptoms of PTSD, such as experiencing painful memories, insomnia and flashbacks. Certain people seem to be especially prone to developing PTSD, including those who receive chemotherapy, and those who develop metastases and symptoms related to their cancer.[106]

People with PTSD often report flashbacks 'out of the blue' and vivid dreams and nightmares about the trauma, such as when they were told they had cancer or it had recurred, pain from the malignancy or its treatment or long stays in hospital. They typically avoid places and people that evoke memories of the cancer, refuse to speak about their experiences and feel constantly on guard or emotionally numb. PTSD can place a considerable strain on relationships and increases the risk of suicide, drug and alcohol abuse and aggression, so speak to your GP or cancer team and get help.

muscles, 'pins and needles' and shortness of breath. Keep a note of when and where the symptoms arise.

Treating anxiety and depression

Begin by trying to identify why you feel anxious or depressed. Try to be specific rather than just saying 'the cancer'. What particularly bothers you? Fear of death? Concerns regarding pain? Worries about recurrence? The impact on your family? Ask yourself what unanswered questions and unresolved issues you have in relation to the cancer and its treatment as both can cause stress and anxiety. Ask your cancer team or a charity for the answers to questions you have about the malignancy and its treatment.

Try to avoid becoming preoccupied with symptoms and watching for signs of recurrence. A stomach ache can still be just indigestion even when you have cancer. Indeed, anxiety can cause muscular aches and pains, which you might worry are signs of recurrence. Also, while carers need to watch for new signs and symptoms, asking too regularly can fuel anxiety.

If anxiety, PTSD or depression interferes with your daily life, speak to your GP or cancer team. They can address particular issues that may cause you to feel anxious, such as poorly controlled pain. They might also suggest antidepressants and anxiolytics. These do not cure depression or anxiety in the way that, for example, antibiotics cure bacterial infections, but might alleviate symptoms, offering you the opportunity to address the causes. Talking treatments often deal with thoughts and behaviours that trigger depression, anxiety or PTSD. In addition, numerous CAMs relieve anxiety, stress and depression. You can find out more in *The Holistic Guide for Cancer Survivors* (see Further reading) or by contacting patient groups.

You could also ask yourself what and who helped you get through difficult times in the past. Who and what made matters worse? You can draw on these resources and insights, which are often more extensive than you realize, to ease you along your cancer journey. Try to take part in more family and recreational activities, which can help take your mind off your troubles. Get out and about in nature, which seems to have an anti-anxiety action in addition to the benefits of exercise. Cut back on caffeine and alcohol, both of which can worsen anxiety. Drinking too much alcohol can also exacerbate depression.

10

What's next?

As mentioned in the Introduction, the cancer journey takes place in broadly three stages.

- Soon after diagnosis, the cancer team tries to cure or limit the damage caused by the malignancy. This might involve surgery, radiotherapy, medicines or, usually, a mixture of approaches.
- During the recovery phase, you get over the worst effects of treatment and restore your physical and mental well-being. The cancer team will monitor you to detect relapses.
- During the maintenance phase, you take steps to prevent or delay a recurrence, prevent additional malignancies and reduce the risk of other preventable diseases, such as a heart attack, osteoporosis and stroke.[6]

This book has focused mainly on the first of these stages. My *The Holistic Guide for Cancer Survivors* (see Further reading) places more emphasis on the second two stages, but this chapter will briefly consider the next steps in the cancer journey. These are only broad outlines – the prognosis varies considerably from person to person.

Palliative care

Despite impressive and continuing advances in treatment, there is, unfortunately, little hope of curing most advanced or metastatic cancers, so your cancer team might offer palliative care. *This does not mean the end of your cancer treatment.* On the contrary, palliative care aims to minimize symptoms, side effects and suffering while optimizing your quality of life, your ability to reach as many of your goals as possible and make the most of your relationships. Palliative care covers your emotional, spiritual, mental and social as well as physical well-being, and evolves as your needs alter. This means that you and your family need to keep the cancer team up to date with how you feel. They will ask, but do not be afraid to be proactive about discussing your symptoms, needs and difficulties before they do.

Depending on your symptoms, general health and well-being, and the type and severity of your side effects, your cancer team might suggest additional 'supportive' treatments. Always tell your GP or cancer team if you experience pain – changing your pain-killers usually helps. If not, cancer medicines, surgery, radiotherapy and other treatments might shrink or remove some metastases that cause pain. The cancer team might suggest drugs to tackle specific symptoms or side effects, such as nausea, diarrhoea or constipation. Never take any medicine – even one generally available without a prescription – without speaking to your cancer team first.

No two people experience advanced cancer in the same way, so doctors and nurses individualize palliative care to meet your wishes and needs. You can, for instance, decide where you would like to receive care – at home, in hospital or in a hospice. This can be flexible – you might consider spending a few days in a hospice to give your carers at home a break. These are important decisions and there is not space to consider palliative care fully here. Speak to your cancer team or contact the cancer charities for more information and help.

Social support

Support from family, friends and other groups can help people adapt to life with cancer. Religious groups offer social and practical as well as spiritual support. A study of 200 people with cancer found that religion provided 'mental support and strength' and increased their confidence that their health will recover. In addition, religion helped people cope with cancer-related stress 'positively and optimistically', reduced anxiety and helped them face uncertainties about the disease's progression.[107]

In another study, researchers analysed 9,267 women's social networks within approximately two years of their being diagnosed with breast cancer. The researchers considered five elements of social networking: spouse or partner; religious ties; community ties; friendships; numbers of living first-degree relatives. Over an average of almost 11 years, socially isolated women were about two-fifths (43 per cent) more likely to experience a recurrence of their breast cancer than socially integrated women. In addition, deaths from breast cancer (64 per cent) and total mortality (69 per cent) were about two-thirds higher and deaths unrelated to breast cancer were more than four-fifths (82 per cent) higher in socially isolated women.[108]

So why does a social network help you cope? Religion, close family and friends can create a sense of community and belonging, which can bolster your mental and physical resources and offer social, practical and emotional support. Your partner's, family's and friends' practical and emotional support can be invaluable if you are, for example, trying to drink less alcohol, quit smoking, take more exercise, change your diet or take medicines as prescribed. Your partner, family and friends can help you adopt a healthy lifestyle, ignore bad moods triggered by the disease or lifestyle changes, boost your motivation, watch out for issues – including fatigue, anxiety and depression – and encourage you to see a doctor when you feel unwell or seem to be taking a turn for the worse or developing side effects.

Develop relationships that preserve or enhance your emotional well-being and bolster your ability to cope; disengage from those that are counterproductive. After all, social networks that cause profound stress are hardly good for your mental or physical health. In some cases, such as your family, you might not be able to remove yourself from the network, but you can probably find ways to limit its negative influence.

Meanwhile, partners, family members and friends need to tread the fine line between 'nagging' – even with the best intentions – and 'support'. Support helps and reinforces their loved one's efforts to tackle unhealthy behaviours. Control – trying to persuade a partner to adopt healthy behaviours when he or she is unwilling or unable – can reduce the likelihood that the person will make the changes and can undermine his or her mental health.

Residual symptoms

Residual symptoms are common among cancer survivors. For example, persistent difficulty swallowing, dry mouth or poor absorption of nutrients can make eating awkward and lead to weight and muscle loss, among other things.[36] A dietician (ask your GP or a cancer team for a referral) can suggest ways to tackle any lingering nutritional difficulties.

Fatigue, depression and other mood disturbances, trouble sleeping, pain and cognitive issues seem to be particularly common among cancer survivors.[90] Indeed, a third of cancer survivors reported that their symptoms were as bad a year after their diagnosis – when they were not receiving treatment – as at the start of their cancer journey.[90] Furthermore, between a fifth and a third of cancer survivors experience fatigue at least five years after their diagnosis or the end of treatment.[90] Some people, for reasons doctors do not fully understand, seem to be especially likely to develop long-term cancer-related fatigue. Urinary, gastrointestinal and sexual symptoms can persist for years after treatment of pelvic cancers ends too. People who survive breast cancer might endure chronic lymphoedema (see page 111).[1]

Sometimes symptoms arise months or even years after treatment ends, such as osteoporosis following endocrine (hormonal) therapies, and heart disease after certain types of chemotherapy or radiotherapy. Similarly, patients less than 40 years old treated with radiotherapy or chemotherapy for Hodgkin's lymphoma, non-Hodgkin's lymphoma or testicular cancer are five times more likely than healthy people to develop congestive heart failure, which typically arises more than ten years after treatment ends.[1]

The long-term psychological effects

Apart from the chronic illnesses caused by the cancer or its treatment, people might experience difficulties dealing with the psychological and emotional fallout from the cancer years later.

Being diagnosed with cancer forces you to confront your mortality, even if the malignancy is not terminal. You might need to adjust your lifestyle or body image – such as following surgery – for the rest of your life. You might need to change or leave employment, especially if you have marked cancer-related fatigue.[90] Not surprisingly, cancer survivors and their families often shoulder a considerable long-term psychological burden.

Fears that the cancer will recur can dominate some survivors' lives after remission. The longer you are cancer free ('in remission'), the more likely it is that you are cured. For most cancers, the risk of recurrence (relapse) is relatively small after remission lasts five years. Nevertheless, cancers occasionally occur long after this. About 1 in 200 breast cancers relapse more than 10 years after the initial diagnosis, for example – one woman had a recurrence of her breast cancer 27 years after the malignancy was first found.[109] Very occasionally, Hodgkin's lymphoma can recur 15–30 years after diagnosis, even following a supposed cure.[2]

It is easy to become preoccupied with watching for signs that the cancer is progressing or recurring. Ironically, this increases the likelihood that you will notice – and worry about – an innocuous symptom. A stomach ache might signal that the cancer has seeded a gastric metastasis – but it is more likely to be indigestion.[83] As mentioned above, anxiety and depression can cause physical symptoms, such as muscle spasms and pain. Equally, though, brain metastases, some medicines and uncontrolled pain can cause anxiety and depression. Essentially, therefore, while you should be vigilant, try not to worry excessively or become preoccupied but also never ignore a change – always check with your cancer team.

Even if you do not need palliative care, managing cancer does not end with the last chemotherapy infusion or the final radiotherapy session. You might need to take medicines for several years, perhaps even the rest of your life, to stop the malignancy recurring. You might experience long-term symptoms or difficulties. You might have to pick up the pieces psychologically after dealing with the diagnosis or the trauma of treatment. You will need to develop a plan individual to you that, typically, includes:[12, 36]

- follow-up visits with your cancer team;
- changes that help you live with or overcome residual symptoms;
- optimizing your general health and lifestyle, including dietary advice to reduce the risk of a recurrence (a personalized dietary and exercise programme can also help rebuild muscle strength and correct symptoms such as anaemia);
- improving your mental and spiritual well-being;
- watching for recurrence and new cancers.

A last word

I will leave the last word to William Osler – one of the greatest doctors in the eighteenth and early nineteenth centuries. Osler reported the case of a patient bedridden with metastatic breast cancer. The malignancy had spread to her spine, other breast and right eye. Two years later, Osler reported: 'She drove a mile and a half to the station to meet me and drove me to the station on my return.' Osler said the case – and others like it – 'are among the most remarkable' in medicine – they illustrate that 'no condition', not even cancer, 'however desperate, is quite hopeless'.[71]

Useful addresses

There are numerous self-help groups for specific cancers. Your cancer team or one of the general charities, such as Cancer Research UK or Macmillan Cancer Support, should be able to put you in touch.

Action Cancer (Northern Ireland)
Action Cancer House
1 Marlborough Park
Belfast
County Antrim BT9 6XS
Tel.: 028 9080 3344
Website: www.actioncancer.org

Action on Smoking and Health (ASH)
Sixth Floor, Suites 59–63
New House
67–68 Hatton Garden
London EC1N 8JY
Tel.: 020 7404 0242
Website: www.ash.org.uk

Alcohol Concern
27 Swinton Street
London WC1X 9NW
Tel.: 020 3907 8480
Website: www.alcoholconcern.org.uk

Alcoholics Anonymous
PO Box 1
10 Toft Green
York YO1 7NJ
Tel.: 0800 9177 650 (helpline)
Website: www.alcoholics-anonymous.org.uk

Breast Cancer Care
Chester House
1–3 Brixton Road
London SW9 6DE
Tel.: 0808 800 6000
Website: www.breastcancercare.org.uk

Breast Cancer UK
BM Box 7767
London WC1N 3XX
Tel.: 0845 680 1322
Website: www.breastcanceruk.org.uk

British Association for Behavioural and Cognitive Psychotherapies (BABCP)
Imperial House
Hornby Street
Bury
Lancashire BL9 5BN
Tel.: 0161 705 4304
Website: www.babcp.com

British Association for Counselling and Psychotherapy (BACP)
BACP House
15 St John's Business Park
Lutterworth
Leicestershire LE17 4HB
Tel.: 01455 883300
Website: www.bacp.co.uk

British Association of Medical Hypnosis (BAMH)
45 Hyde Park Square
London W2 2JT
Tel.: 07711 681134
Website: www.bamh.org.uk

British Dietetic Association (BDA)
5th Floor, Charles House
148/9 Great Charles Street
Queensway
Birmingham B3 3HT
Tel.: 0121 200 8080
Website: www.bda.uk.com

British Liver Trust
6 Dean Park Crescent
Bournemouth BH1 1HL
Tel.: 0800 652 7330 (helpline)
Website: www.britishlivertrust.org.uk

Cancer Research UK
PO Box 1561
Oxford OX4 9GZ
Tel.: 0300 123 1022
Website: www.cancerresearchuk.org

Child Bereavement UK
Clare Charity Centre
Wycombe Road
Saunderton
Buckinghamshire HP14 4BF
Tel.: 01494 568900
Website: www.childbereavementuk.org

Complementary and Natural Healthcare Council (CNHC)
46–48 East Smithfield
London E1W 1AW
Tel.: 020 3668 0406
Website: www.cnhc.org.uk

Confederation of Healing Organizations, Institute for Complementary and Natural Medicine and British Register of Complementary Practitioners
Email: office@brcp.uk
Tel.: 0300 302 0715
Website: www.icnm.org.uk

Cruse Bereavement Care
PO Box 800
Richmond
Surrey TW9 1RG
Tel.: 0808 808 1677 (helpline)
Website: www.cruse.org.uk

Federation of Holistic Therapists (FHT)
18 Shakespeare Business Centre
Hathaway Close
Eastleigh SO50 4SR
Tel.: 023 8062 4350
Website: www.fht.org.uk

General Regulatory Council for Complementary Therapies (GRCCT)
Box 437, Office 6
Slington House
Rankine Road
Basingstoke RG24 8PH
Tel.: 0870 314 4031
Website: www.grcct.org

Health and Care Professions Council (HCPC)
Park House
184 Kennington Park Road
London SE11 4BU
Tel.: 0300 500 6184
Website: www.hpc-uk.co.uk

Leukaemia Care
One Birch Court
Blackpole East
Worcester WR3 8SG
Tel.: 08088 010 444 (helpline)
Website: www.leukaemiacare.org.uk

Lymphoma Association
3 Cromwell Court
New Street
Aylesbury HP20 2PB
Tel.: 0808 808 5555 (helpline)
Website: www.lymphomas.org.uk

Macmillan Cancer Support
89 Albert Embankment
London SE1 7UQ
Tel.: 0808 808 00 00 (helpline)
Website: www.macmillan.org.uk

Marie Curie
89 Albert Embankment
London SE1 7TP
Tel.: 0800 090 2309 (helpline)
Website: www.mariecurie.org.uk

Orchid (male cancers)
231–233 North Gower Street
London NW1 2NR
Tel.: 0808 802 0010 (helpline)
Website: https://orchid-cancer.org.uk

Prostate Cancer UK
Fourth floor
The Counting House
53 Tooley Street
London SE1 2QN
Tel.: 0800 074 8383 (helpline)
Website: https://prostatecanceruk.org

Rarer Cancers Foundation
Unit 7B, Evelyn Court
Grinstead Road
London SE8 5AD
Tel.: 0800 334 5551 (helpline)
Website: http://rarercancers.org.uk

Roy Castle Lung Cancer Foundation
The Roy Castle Centre
4–6 Enterprise Way
Wavertree Technology Park
Liverpool L13 1FB
Tel.: 0333 323 7200
Website: www.roycastle.org

Teenage Cancer Trust
Third floor
93 Newman Street
London W1T 3EZ
Tel.: 020 7612 0370
Website: www.teenagecancertrust.org

Tenovus Cancer Care
Gleider House
Ty Glas Road
Cardiff CF14 5BD
Tel.: 0808 808 1010 (helpline)
Website: www.tenovuscancercare.org.uk

References

1 Rubin, G., Berendsen, A., Crawford, S. M., Dommett, R., Earle, C., Emery, J., Fahey, T., Grassi, L., Grunfeld, E., Gupta, S., Hamilton, W., Hiom, S., Hunter, D., Lyratzopoulos, G., Macleod, U., Mason, R., Mitchell, G., Neal, R. D., Peake, M., Roland, M., Seifert, B., Sisler, J., Sussman, J., Taplin, S., Vedsted, P., Voruganti, T., Walter, F., Wardle, J., Watson, E., Weller, D., Wender, R., Whelan, J., Whitlock, J., Wilkinson, C., de Wit, N. and Zimmermann, C. (2015) 'The expanding role of primary care in cancer control', *The Lancet Oncology*, 16:1231–72.

2 Bower, M. and Waxman, J. (2015) *Oncology: Lecture notes*. Chichester: Wiley.

3 Palmieri, C., Bird, E. and Simcock, R. (2013) *ABC of Cancer Care*. Chichester: Wiley-Blackwell and BMJ Books.

4 Smittenaar, C. R., Petersen, K. A., Stewart, K. and Moitt, N. (2016) 'Cancer incidence and mortality projections in the UK until 2035', *British Journal of Cancer*, 115:1147–55.

5 Tabernero, J., Vyas, M., Giuliani, R., Arnold, D., Cardoso, F., Casali, P. G., Cervantes, A., Eggermont, A. M., Eniu, A., Jassem, J., Pentheroudakis, G., Peters, S., Rauh, S., Zielinski, C. C., Stahel, R. A., Voest, E., Douillard, J.-Y., McGregor, K. and Ciardiello, F. (2017) 'Biosimilars: A position paper of the European Society for Medical Oncology, with particular reference to oncology prescribers', *ESMO Open*, 1(6) e000142.

6 Brown, J., Byers, T., Thompson, K., Eldridge, B., Doyle, C. and Williams, A. M. (2001) 'Nutrition during and after cancer treatment: A guide for informed choices by cancer survivors', *CA: A Cancer Journal for Clinicians*, 51:153–81.

7 Schrijver, K. and Schrijver, I. (2015) *Living with the Stars*. Oxford: Oxford University Press.

8 Cooper, C. (2016) *Blood: A very short introduction*. Oxford: Oxford University Press.

9 Williams, G. H. and Stoeber, K. (2012) 'The cell cycle and cancer', *The Journal of Pathology*, 226:352–64.

10 Armstrong, S. (2015) *p53: The Gene that Cracked the Cancer Code*. London: Bloomsbury.

11 Masters, J. R. (2002) 'HeLa cells 50 years on: The good, the bad and the ugly', *Nature Reviews Cancer*, 2:315–19.

12 Saunders, C. and Jassal, S. (2009) *Breast Cancer: The facts*. Oxford: Oxford University Press.

13 Riley, T. R., 3rd and Bhatti, A. M. (2001) 'Preventive strategies in chronic liver disease: Part I. Alcohol, vaccines, toxic medications and supplements, diet and exercise', *American Family Physician*, 64:1555–60.

14 Javier, R. T. and Butel, J. S. (2008) 'The history of tumor virology', *Cancer Research*, 68:7693–706.

15 Cancer (2012) 'Genome Atlas Network: Comprehensive molecular portraits of human breast tumours', *Nature*, 490:61–70.

16 James, N. (2011) *Cancer: A very short introduction.* Oxford: Oxford University Press.

17 Mukherjee, M. (2011) *The Emperor of All Maladies: A biography of cancer.* London: Fourth Estate.

18 Kuru, B., Camlibel, M., Dinc, S., Gulcelik, M. A., Gonullu, D. and Alagol, H. (2008) 'Prognostic factors for survival in breast cancer patients who developed distant metastasis subsequent to definitive surgery', *Singapore Medical Journal*, 49:904–11.

19 Greener, M. (2014) 'Tackling HPV and cervical cancer: Looking at the whole picture', *British Journal of School Nursing*, 9:377–80.

20 Matsumoto, K., Oki, A., Furuta, R., Maeda, H., Yasugi, T., Takatsuka, N., Mitsuhashi, A., Fujii, T., Hirai, Y., Iwasaka, T., Yaegashi, N., Watanabe, Y., Nagai, Y., Kitagawa, T., Yoshikawa, H., Japan HPV and Cervical Cancer Study Group (2011) 'Predicting the progression of cervical precursor lesions by human papillomavirus genotyping: A prospective cohort study', *International Journal of Cancer*, 128:2898–910.

21 Hajdu, S. I. (2012) 'A note from history: Landmarks in history of cancer, part 4', *Cancer*, 118:4914–28.

22 Parkin, D. M. and Darby, S. C. (2011) 'Cancers in 2010 attributable to ionising radiation exposure in the UK', *British Journal of Cancer*, 105:S57–S65.

23 Parkin, D. M., Boyd, L. and Walker, L. C. (2011) 'The fraction of cancer attributable to lifestyle and environmental factors in the UK in 2010', *British Journal of Cancer*, 105:S77–S81.

24 Ryndock, E. J. and Meyers, C. (2014) 'A risk for non-sexual transmission of human papillomavirus?', *Expert Review of Anti-infective Therapy*, 12:1165–70.

25 Powell, N., Cuschieri, K., Cubie, H., Hibbitts, S., Rosillon, D., De Souza, S. C., Molijn, A., Quint, W., Holl, K. and Fiander, A. (2013) 'Cervical cancers associated with human papillomavirus types 16, 18 and 45 are diagnosed in younger women than cancers associated with other types: A cross-sectional observational study in Wales and Scotland (UK)', *Journal of Clinical Virology*, 58:571–4.

26 Deligeoroglou, E., Giannouli, A., Athanasopoulos, N., Karountzos, V., Vatopoulou, A., Dimopoulos, K. and Creatsas, G. (2013) 'HPV infection: immunological aspects and their utility in future therapy', *Infectious Diseases in Obstetric Gynecology*, 2013:540850.

27 Anderson, T. A., Schick, V., Herbenick, D., Dodge, B. and Fortenberry, J. D. (2014) 'A study of human papillomavirus on vaginally inserted sex toys, before and after cleaning, among women who have sex with women and men', *Sexually Transmitted Infections*, 90:529–31.

28 King, E. M., Gilson, R., Beddows, S., Soldan, K., Panwar, K., Young, C.,

Jit, M., Edmunds, W. J. and Sonnenberg, P. (2015) 'Oral human papillomavirus (HPV) infection in men who have sex with men: Prevalence and lack of anogenital concordance', *Sexually Transmitted Infections*, 91:284–6.

29 Delere, Y., Wichmann, O., Klug, S. J., van der Sande, M., Terhardt, M., Zepp, F. and Harder, T. (2014) 'The efficacy and duration of vaccine protection against human papillomavirus: A systematic review and meta-analysis', *Deutsches Ärzteblatt International*, 111:584–91.

30 Bae, J.-M. and Kim, E. H. (2016) 'Epstein-Barr virus and gastric cancer risk: A meta-analysis with meta-regression of case-control studies', *Journal of Preventive Medicine and Public Health*, 49:97–107.

31 Norat, T., Aune, D., Chan, D. and Romaguera, D. (2014) 'Fruits and vegetables: Updating the epidemiologic evidence for the WCRF/AICR lifestyle recommendations for cancer prevention', in Zappia, V. et al. (eds), *Advances in Nutrition and Cancer*. Berlin, Heidelberg: Springer. Pp. 35–50.

32 Kenfield, S. A., Batista, J. L., Jahn, J. L., Downer, M. K., Van Blarigan, E. L., Sesso, H. D., Giovannucci, E. L., Stampfer, M. J. and Chan, J. M. (2015) 'Development and application of a lifestyle score for prevention of lethal prostate cancer', *Journal of the National Cancer Institute*, 108:pii: djv329.

33 Yang, M., Kenfield, S. A., Van Blarigan, E. L., Batista, J. L., Sesso, H. D., Ma, J., Stampfer, M. J. and Chavarro, J. E. (2015) 'Dietary patterns after prostate cancer diagnosis in relation to disease-specific and total mortality', *Cancer Prevention Research*, 8:545–51.

34 Cancer Research UK and UK Health Forum (2016) 'Short and sweet: Why the government should introduce a sugary drinks tax'. Available online at: <www.ukhealthforum.org.uk/who-we-are/our-work/modelling/publications/?entryid43=54920>.

35 Parkin, D. M. and Boyd, L. (2011) 'Cancers attributable to overweight and obesity in the UK in 2010', *British Journal of Cancer*, 105:S34–S37.

36 Brown, J., Byers, T., Thompson, K., Eldridge, B., Doyle, C. and Williams, A. M. (2001) 'Nutrition during and after cancer treatment: A guide for informed choices by cancer survivors', *CA: A Cancer Journal for Clinicians*, 51:153–181.

37 Nelson, D. E., Jarman, D. W., Rehm, J., Greenfield, T. K., Rey, G., Kerr, W. C., Miller, P., Shield, K. D., Ye, Y. and Naimi, T. S. (2013) 'Alcohol-attributable cancer deaths and years of potential life lost in the United States', *American Journal of Public Health*, 103:641–8.

38 Miller, P. M., Day, T. A. and Ravenel, M. C. (2006) 'Clinical implications of continued alcohol consumption after diagnosis of upper aerodigestive tract cancer', *Alcohol and Alcoholism*, 41:140–2.

39 Parkin, D. M. (2011) 'Tobacco-attributable cancer burden in the UK in 2010', *British Journal of Cancer*, 105:S6–S13.

40 Inoue-Choi, M., Liao, L. M., Reyes-Guzman, C., Hartge, P., Caporaso, N. and Freedman, N. D. (2017) 'Association of long-term, low-

intensity smoking with all-cause and cause-specific mortality in the National Institutes of Health–AARP diet and health study', *JAMA Internal Medicine*, 177:87–95.

41 Danson, S., Rowland, C., Rowe, R., Ellis, S., Crabtree, C., Horsman, J., Wadsley, J., Hatton, M., Woll, P. and Eiser, C. (2016) 'The relationship between smoking and quality of life in advanced lung cancer patients: a prospective longitudinal study', *Supportive Care in Cancer*, 24:1507–16.

42 Baser, S., Shannon, V. R., Eapen, G. A., Jimenez, C. A., Onn, A., Lin, E. and Morice, R. C. (2006) 'Smoking cessation after diagnosis of lung cancer is associated with a beneficial effect on performance status', *Chest*, 130:1784–90.

43 Montgomery, G. H., Schnur, J. B. and Kravits, K. (2013) 'Hypnosis for cancer care: Over 200 years young', *CA: A Cancer Journal for Clinicians*, 63:31–44.

44 Annunziato, A. (2008) 'DNA packaging: nucleosomes and chromatin', *Nature Education*, 1:26. Available online at: <www.nature.com./scitable/topicpage/dna-packaging-nucleosomes-and-chromatin-310>

45 Cybulski, C., Nazarali, S. and Narod, S. A. (2014) 'Multiple primary cancers as a guide to heritability', *International Journal of Cancer*, 135:1756–63.

46 Mei, L., Du, W. and Ma, W. W. (2016) 'Targeting stromal microenvironment in pancreatic ductal adenocarcinoma: controversies and promises', *Journal of Gastrointestinal Oncology*, 7:487–94.

47 Tomasetti, C., Li, L. and Vogelstein, B. (2017) 'Stem cell divisions, somatic mutations, cancer etiology, and cancer prevention', *Science*, 355:1330–4.

48 Friedenson, B. (2005) 'BRCA1 and BRCA2 pathways and the risk of cancers other than breast or ovarian', *Medscape General Medicine*, 7:60.

49 Baker, S. G. (2014) 'A cancer theory kerfuffle can lead to new lines of research', *Journal of the National Cancer Institute*, 107:pii: dju405.

50 Badenhorst, J., Husband, A., Ling, J., Lindsey, L., Todd, A. and Baer, M. (2014) 'Do patients with cancer alarm symptoms present at the community pharmacy?', *International Journal of Pharmacy Practice*, 22 (suppl. 2):32.

51 Borghesi, M., Ahmed, H., Nam, R., Schaeffer, E., Schiavina, R., Taneja, S., Weidner, W. and Loeb, S. (2017) 'Complications after systematic, random, and image-guided prostate biopsy', *European Urology*, 71:353–65.

52 Gaylis, F., Nasseri, R., Fink, L., Calabrese, R., Dato, P. and Cohen, E. (2016) 'Prostate biopsy complications: A dual analysis', *Urology*, 93:135–40.

53 Ellinger, S. (2013) 'Micronutrients, arginine, and glutamine: Does supplementation provide an efficient tool for prevention and treatment of different kinds of wounds?', *Advances in Wound Care*, 3:691–707.

54 Lindley, R. (2008) *Stroke: The facts.* Oxford: Oxford University Press.

55 Kumar, S., Selim, M. H. and Caplan, L. R. (2010) 'Medical complications after stroke', *The Lancet Neurology*, 9:105–18.

56 Anonymous (1996) 'Chapter 2: The development of radiotherapy: physics, technology, methods', *Acta Oncologica*, 35:24–30.

57 Anonymous (1960) 'Obituary: E. H. Grubbé, MD, FACP', *British Medical Journal*, 2:609.

58 Tanderup, K., Ménard, C., Polgar, C., Lindegaard, J. C., Kirisits, C. and Pötter, R. (2017) 'Advancements in brachytherapy', *Advanced Drug Delivery Reviews*, 109:15–25.

59 Scott, A. (2015) 'Non-sting barrier cream in radiotherapy-induced skin reactions', *British Journal of Nursing*, 24:S32, S34–7.

60 Travis, L. B. (2006) 'The epidemiology of second primary cancers', *Cancer Epidemiology Biomarkers & Prevention*, 15:2020–6.

61 Taylor, C., Correa, C., Duane, F. K., Aznar, M. C., Anderson, S. J., Bergh, J., Dodwell, D., Ewertz, M., Gray, R., Jagsi, R., Pierce, L., Pritchard, K. I., Swain, S., Wang, Z., Wang, Y., Whelan, T., Peto, R. and McGale, P. (2017) 'Estimating the risks of breast cancer radiotherapy: Evidence from modern radiation doses to the lungs and heart and from previous randomized trials', *Journal of Clinical Oncology*, 35:1641–9.

62 Tannock, I. F., de Wit, R., Berry, W. R., Horti, J., Pluzanska, A., Chi, K. N., Oudard, S., Théodore, C., James, N. D., Turesson, I., Rosenthal, M. A. and Eisenberger, M. A. (2004) 'Docetaxel plus prednisone or mitoxantrone plus prednisone for advanced prostate cancer', *New England Journal of Medicine*, 351:1502–12.

63 Khoja, L., McGurk, A., O'Hara, C., Chow, S. and Hasan, J. (2015) 'Mortality within 30 days following systemic anti-cancer therapy: A review of all cases over a 4 year period in a tertiary cancer centre', *European Journal of Cancer*, 51:233–40.

64 Silverman, R., Smith, L. and Sundar, S. (2014) 'Benchmarking 30 day mortality after palliative chemotherapy for solid tumours', *Clinical Oncology*, 26:236.

65 Karagöz Özen, D. S., Ozturk, M. A., Aydin, Ö., Turna, Z. H., Ilvan, S. and Özüroglu, M. (2014) 'Receptor expression discrepancy between primary and metastatic breast cancer lesions', *Oncology Research and Treatment*, 37:622–6.

66 Roth, M. Y. and Amory, J. K. (2016) 'Beyond the condom: Frontiers in male contraception', *Seminars in Reproductive Medicine*, 34:183–90.

67 Sam, A. and Meeran, K. (2009) *Lecture Notes in Endocrinology and Diabetes*. Oxford: Wiley-Blackwell.

68 Komatsu, H., Yagasaki, K., Yamauchi, H., Yamauchi, T. and Takebayashi, T. (2016) 'A self-directed home yoga programme for women with breast cancer during chemotherapy: A feasibility study', *International Journal of Nursing Practice*, 22:258–66.

69 Atkins, L. and Fallowfield, L. (2006) 'Intentional and non-intentional non-adherence to medication amongst breast cancer patients', *European Journal of Cancer*, 42:2271–6.

70 Ito, E., Nakano, S., Otsuka, M., Mibu, A., Karikomi, M., Oinuma, T. and Yamamoto, M. (2016) 'Spontaneous breast cancer remission: A case report', *International Journal of Surgery Case Reports*, 25:132–6.

71 Papac, R. (1996) 'Spontaneous regression of cancer', *Cancer Treatment Reviews*, 22:395–423.

72 Ventegodt, S., Jacobsen, S. and Merrick, J. (2009) 'Clinical holistic medicine: A case of induced spontaneous remission in a patient with non-Hodgkin b-lymphoma', *Journal of Alternative Medcine Research*, 1:101–10.

73 Horii, R., Akiyama, F., Kasumi, F., Koike, M. and Sakamoto, G. (2005) 'Spontaneous "healing" of breast cancer', *Breast Cancer*, 12:140–4.

74 Donnelly, L. (2015) '"Cure for terminal cancer" found in game-changing drugs', *Daily Telegraph*. Available online at: <www.telegraph.co.uk/news/health/news/11641771/Cure-for-terminal-cancer-found-in-game-changing-drugs.html>

75 Gorman, C. (2015) 'Cancer Immunotherapy: The cutting edge gets sharper', *Scientific American*. Available online at: <www.scientificamerican.com/article/cancer-immunotherapy-the-cutting-edge-gets-sharper>

76 Greener, M. (2016) 'Cancer immunotherapy: Should we believe the hype?', *Prescriber*, 27:13–20.

77 Pieters, T. (1993) 'Interferon and its first clinical trial: Looking behind the scenes', *Medical History*, 37:270–95.

78 Wiemann, B. and Starnes, C. O. (1994) 'Coley's toxins, tumor necrosis factor and cancer research: A historical perspective', *Pharmacology & Therapeutics*, 64:529–64.

79 Farkona, S., Diamandis, E. P. and Blasutig, I. M. (2016) 'Cancer immunotherapy: The beginning of the end of cancer?', *BMC Medicine*, 14:1–18.

80 Bracci, L., Schiavoni, G., Sistigu, A. and Belardelli, F. (2014) 'Immune-based mechanisms of cytotoxic chemotherapy: Implications for the design of novel and rationale-based combined treatments against cancer', *Cell Death and Differentiation*, 21:15–25.

81 El-Osta, H., Shahid, K., Mills, G. M. and Peddi, P. (2016) 'Immune checkpoint inhibitors: The new frontier in non-small-cell lung cancer treatment', *Onco Targets and Therapy*, 9:5101–16.

82 Kravits, K. G. (2015) 'Hypnosis for the management of anticipatory nausea and vomiting', *Journal of the Advanced Practitioner in Oncology*, 6:225–9.

83 Chochinov, H. and Breitbart, W. (eds) (2009) *Handbook of Psychiatry in Palliative Medicine*. Oxford: Oxford University Press.

84 Hammer, M. J., Ercolano, E. A., Wright, F., Dickson, V. V., Chyun, D. and Melkus, G. D. E. (2015) 'Self-management for adult patients with cancer: an integrative review', *Cancer Nursing*, 38:E10–E26.

85 Malton, S. (2015) 'Managing chemo side-effects', *Pharmacy Magazine*, June:16.

86 Ben-Arye, E., Polliack, A., Schiff, E., Tadmor, T. and Samuels, N. (2013) 'Advising patients on the use of non-herbal nutritional supplements during cancer therapy: A need for doctor–patient communication', *Journal of Pain and Symptom Management*, 46:887–96.

87 Newton, S., Hickey, M. and Marrs, J. (2009) *Mosby's Oncology Nursing Advisor: A comprehensive guide to clinical practice*. St. Louis, MO and London: Mosby.

88 Armstrong, L. E., Ganio, M. S., Casa, D. J., Lee, E. C., McDermott, B. P., Klau, J. F., Jimenez, L., Le Bellego, L., Chevillotte, E. and Lieberman, H. R. (2012) 'Mild dehydration affects mood in healthy young women', *The Journal of Nutrition*, 142:382–8.

89 Ganio, M. S., Armstrong, L. E., Casa, D. J., McDermott, B. P., Lee, E. C., Yamamoto, L. M., Marzano, S., Lopez, R. M., Jimenez, L., Le Bellego, L., Chevillotte, E. and Lieberman, H. R. (2011) 'Mild dehydration impairs cognitive performance and mood of men', *British Journal of Nutrition*, 106:1535–43.

90 Wu, H.-S. and Harden, J. K. (2015) 'Symptom burden and quality of life in survivorship: A review of the literature', *Cancer Nursing*, 38:E29–E54.

91 Priestman, T. (2007) *Coping with Radiotherapy*. London: Sheldon Press.

92 Battaglini, C. L., Mills, R. C., Phillips, B. L., Lee, J. T., Story, C. E., Nascimento, M. G. B. and Hackney, A. C. (2014) 'Twenty-five years of research on the effects of exercise training in breast cancer survivors: A systematic review of the literature', *World Journal of Clinical Oncology*, 5:177–90.

93 Borch, K. B., Braaten, T., Lund, E. and Weiderpass, E. (2015) 'Physical activity before and after breast cancer diagnosis and survival: The Norwegian women and cancer cohort study', *BMC Cancer*, 15:1–10.

94 Sutton, A., Crew, A. and Wysong, A. (2016) 'Redefinition of skin cancer as a chronic disease', *JAMA Dermatology*, 152:255–6.

95 Hofbauer, K., Anker, S., Inui, A. and Nicholson, J. (2005) *Pharmacotherapy of Cachexia*. Boca Raton, FL and London: CRC Press.

96 Gamper, E.-M., Zabernigg, A., Wintner, L. M., Giesinger, J. M., Oberguggenberger, A., Kemmler, G., Sperner-Unterweger, B. and Holzner, B. (2012) 'Coming to your senses: Detecting taste and smell alterations in chemotherapy patients: A systematic review', *Journal of Pain and Symptom Management*, 44:880–95.

97 Ijpma, I., Renken, R. J., ter Horst, G. J. and Reyners, A. K. L. (2015) 'Metallic taste in cancer patients treated with chemotherapy', *Cancer Treatment Reviews*, 41:179–86.

98 Garland, S. N., Xie, S. X., Li, Q., Seluzicki, C., Basal, C. and Mao, J. J. (2017) 'Comparative effectiveness of electro-acupuncture versus gabapentin for sleep disturbances in breast cancer survivors with hot flashes: A randomized trial', *Menopause*, 24:517–23.

99 Wiśniewska, I., Jochymek, B., Lenart-Lipińska, M. and Chabowski, M. (2016) 'The pharmacological and hormonal therapy of hot flushes in breast cancer survivors', *Breast Cancer*, 23:178–82.

100 Chao, J. H. and Page, S. T. (2016) 'The current state of male hormonal contraception', *Pharmacology & Therapeutics*, 163:109–17.

101 Dautricourt, S., Marzloff, V. and Dollfus, S. (2015) 'Meningiomatosis revealed by a major depressive syndrome', *BMJ Case Reports*, 2015:Doi:10.1136/bcr-2015-211909.

102 Tylee, A. and Gandhi, P. (2005) 'The importance of somatic symptoms in depression in primary care', *The Primary Care Companion for CNS Disorders*, 7:167–76.

103 Edwards, V. (2003) *Depression: What you really need to know*. London: Robinson.

104 Russell, A. (2009) *The Social Basis of Medicine* (1st edn). Oxford: Wiley-Blackwell.

105 Hoge, E. A., Ivkovic, A. and Fricchione, G. L. (2012) 'Generalized anxiety disorder: Diagnosis and treatment', *BMJ*, 345:e7500.

106 Lin, Y.-H., Kao, C.-C., Wu, S.-F., Hung, S.-L., Yang, H.-Y. and Tung, H.-Y. (2017) 'Risk factors of post-traumatic stress symptoms in patients with cancer', *Journal of Clinical Nursing*, 26:3137–43.

107 Tsai, T. J., Chung, U. L., Chang, C. J. and Wang, H. H. (2016) 'Influence of religious beliefs on the health of cancer patients', *Asian Pacific Journal of Cancer Prevention*, 17:2315–20.

108 Kroenke, C. H., Michael, Y. L., Poole, E. M., Kwan, M. L., Nechuta, S., Leas, E., Caan, B. J., Pierce, J., Shu, X.-O., Zheng, Y. and Chen, W. Y. (2016) 'Postdiagnosis social networks and breast cancer mortality in the After Breast Cancer Pooling Project', *Cancer*, 123:1228–37.

109 Durdu Keskin, O., Kertmen, N., Karakas, Y., Babacan, T., Arik, Z., Altundag, K. and Gullu, I. (2015) 'A systemic late recurrence after the first operation in a patient diagnosed with early-stage breast cancer: The latest recurrence in the literature', *Journal of BUON*, 20:348.

Further reading

Armstrong, Sue (2015) *p53: The gene that cracked the cancer code*. London: Bloomsbury.

Ausubel, Kenny (2000) *When Healing Becomes a Crime: The amazing story of the Hoxsey Cancer Clinics and the return of alternative therapies*. Rochester, VT: Healing Arts Press.

Bower, Mark and Waxman, Jonathan (2015) *Oncology: Lecture notes*. Chichester: Wiley.

Freeman, Jane (2012) *How to Eat Well When You Have Cancer*. London: Sheldon Press.

Greener, Mark (2013) *Coping with Liver Disease*. London: Sheldon Press.

Greener, Mark (2013) *The Holistic Health Handbook*. London: Sheldon Press.

Greener, Mark (2014) *Coping with Thyroid Disease*. London: Sheldon Press.

Greener, Mark (2015) *Depression and Anxiety: The drug-free way*. London: Sheldon Press.

Greener, Mark (2016) *The Holistic Guide for Cancer Survivors*. London: Sheldon Press.

James, Nicholas (2011) *Cancer: A very short introduction*. Oxford: Oxford University Press.

Krementsov, Nikolai (2004) *The Cure: A story of cancer and politics from the annals of the Cold War*. Chicago: University of Chicago Press.

Mukherjee, Siddhartha (2011) *The Emperor of All Maladies: A biography of cancer*. London: Fourth Estate.

Palmieri, Carlo, Bird, Esther and Simcock, Richard (2013) *ABC of Cancer Care*. Chichester: Wiley-Blackwell and BMJ Books.

Styron, William (1991) *Darkness Visible*. London: Jonathan Cape.

Index